AN OPPORTUNITY FOR A FULL LIFE

AN INTRODUCTION TO ANTHROPOSOPHICAL SOCIAL THERAPY

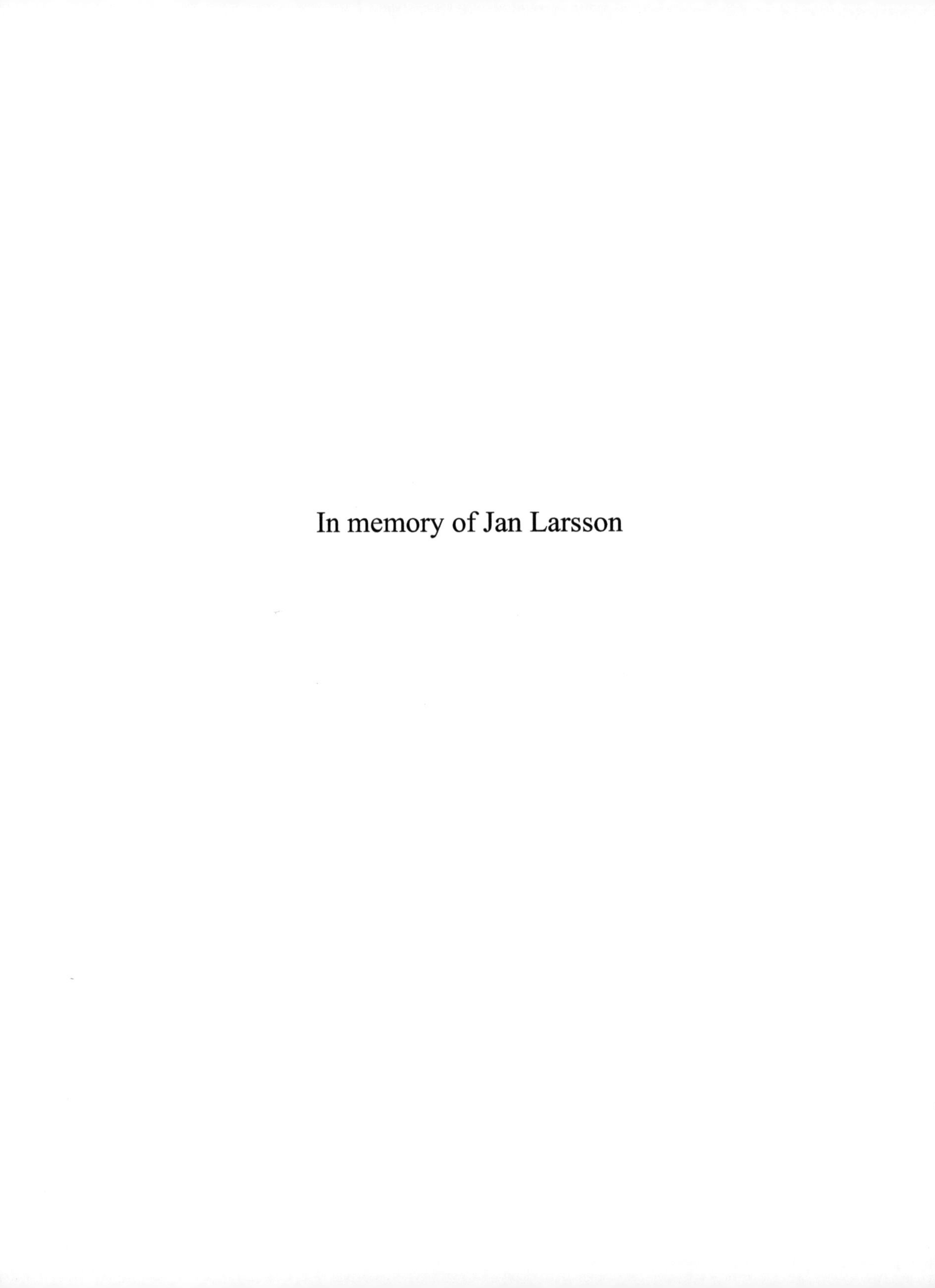

In memory of Jan Larsson

AN OPPORTUNITY FOR A FULL LIFE

AN INTRODUCTION TO ANTHROPOSOPHICAL SOCIAL THERAPY

Sara Sörgärde Siegers

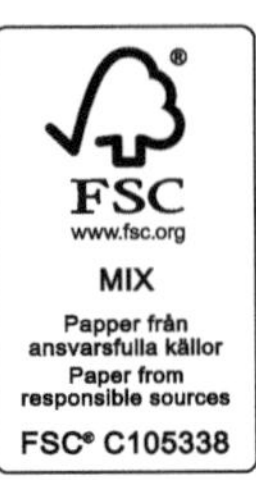

Original title: Möjlighet till ett rikt liv,

Translation and editing: Edeline LeFevre

Illustration: Sara Sörgärde Siegers

Publisher: BoD · Books on Demand, Stockholm, Sweden
Print: Libri Plureos GmbH, Hamburg, Germany

ISBN: 978-91-8080-015-0

CONTENT

FOREWORD

This book came about because I was unable to have an overview and introduction to anthroposophical social therapy. Much of the anthroposophical literature already in existence, at least in Sweden, is written based on work with children and adolescents, which is somewhat different from working with adults. It is also quite difficult to read if you do not have prior knowledge. I missed a first, easier book to put into the hands of an interested co-worker and say, "Here, start with this!".

The idea of this book is for you to get an introduction to some of the most common social therapeutic and anthroposophical concepts. My hope is that you will understand the basics of anthroposophy and social therapy and will be curious to find out more. It will all be presented in simple language, as simple as possible.

Social therapy as based on anthroposophy is complementary to up-to-date knowledge of adults with disabilities rather than being an alternative for it. This means that we work with theories and methods based on modern research and guidelines permeated with knowledge from the anthroposophical view of humanity. Social therapy is very much about how we relate to what we do. As a social therapist you need to develop the ability to see the individual but also to have the knowledge and skills to be able to meet each single person's needs.

> *"Social therapy is not a healing pedagogy. It aims to provide opportunities for adults with disabilities to find social contexts which support body, mind and spirit – through adapted forms of housing, adequate work opportunities, medical therapies, public education and appropriate leisure activities. "*
> Tommy Sydhagen, LäS 12/2009 p23.

This book is a sketchy and comprehensive picture of my own interpretation of social therapy. It is based on various writings, lectures by and conversations with experienced social therapists, as well as on my own experience. All eventual misconceptions are my own.

Sara Sörgärde Siegers

Additional forewords to the English translation

When translating the book, I have come to realise one thing. It is way harder than one may think. Not only do the words need to be translated, but the different social settings need to be addressed somehow as well. There are a few people that have helped me during work on the translation, and for this I am very grateful. First, Karen Rieman that worked hard on the German translation and thereby made the translation into English much easier. Second, a big thank you to Edeline LeFevre who took on the work of translation and editing of the English version.

In the work of translating this book we made some changes to the chapters in the background. We removed some parts that were only relevant for Swedish readers and added new parts about the international work to the translated book.

Since I wrote the original book, I have made new realisations and learned a lot more about Social Therapy and Anthroposophy. I have decided to keep the translation close to the original and not fall into the temptation of rewriting the whole book. That might be a project for the future.

Sara Sörgärde Siegers

BACKGROUND

ANTHROPOSOPHY

"Anthroposophy is a path of knowledge that wants to bring the spiritual in man to the spiritual in the universe", Rudolf Steiner, 1924. (Steiner, 1978 p. 15)

The word anthroposophy comes from the Greek Anthropos – human being, and Sophia - wisdom. Freely translated: How to be a human being. It is a philosophy of life addressing existential questions with a focus on the general human being and what it means to be human. The basic idea of anthroposophy is that the world comprises more than what we can see and touch. There is a spiritual dimension which cannot be explored and explained solely by the usual scientific methods. Anthroposophy was originally developed by Rudolf Steiner.

The task of the human being is to think and acquire knowledge based on freedom, and to constantly develop oneself. We have a responsibility as human beings to ourselves, to each other and to the world we live in. Because of this it will become important to think in a more broadly environmental way, for instance by choosing food which provides good nutrition to the body; food which is produced without toxins and in balance with nature. It then also What kind of environment we surround ourselves with and what kind of materials we use for our clothing is just as important. Yet not only the physicality that surrounds us is important. Working with yourself and your own development and reflecting on yourself as a person and what is the meaning of life are intrinsic aspects.

In anthroposophy, the world is seen as part of a much larger context in that the soul and the self live on even when the body dies. Anthroposophy wants to combine science and human experience with spiritual research in an interdisciplinary way.

The question often comes up whether anthroposophy is a sect, which it is not. The fundamental idea of anthroposophy is very far from that of a sect because it is based on the free will of the human being: every human being has the ability and responsibility to think for themselves. Anthroposophy is not a religion either although it uses Christian concepts and is based on a Christian worldview, yet it is also possible to recognize ideas from other religions and philosophies. It is simply a philosophy of life which can be applied regardless of which religion one belongs to.

Anyone can be an anthroposophist and to become an anthroposophist it is enough to have the earnest intent to do so. When you then study anthroposophical knowledge, you soon realize that you need to actively work on yourself spiritually, soul-wise and physically.

Rudolf Steiner

1861-1925

Rudolf Steiner is the founder of anthroposophy. He was born in Donji Kraljevec in Austria-Hungary in 1861 (today it is in North Croatia), the son of a railway official. He studied mathematics, physics, biology, literature, chemistry, history, and philosophy at the Vienna University of Technology. In 1891 he did his thesis on epistemological issues. In addition, he published many different books and articles in areas such as philosophy and pedagogy. One of his most famous works is the book The Philosophy of Freedom which was published in 1893.

Even as a child, Steiner had supernatural experiences, which he didn't talk about at the time. As an adult, Rudolf Steiner joined the Theosophical Society, but later broke away from it and subsequently founded the Anthroposophical Society. The anthroposophical image of the human being assumes that the soul-spiritual and physical-material are constantly working together. According to Steiner himself, anthroposophy is "a path of knowledge that wants to bring the spiritual in the human being to the spiritual in the universe" (Steiner, 1974 p.15). Steiner wanted to show that research in the supernatural had the same value as the modern science of the body and human biology, that the limit of knowledge can be exceeded while maintaining scientific rigour. Boundaries exist only for the individual, but anyone can move them and expand their field of knowledge.

Many people turned to Rudolf Steiner for advice and to ask him to develop his thoughts on various subjects. He gave lectures and most of the original literature by Rudolf Steiner consists of transcriptions of these lectures. Perhaps this is why they can be difficult to read and understand. In the development of the practical branches of activity, he himself did not do everything, but people close to him developed the practice based on his ideas.

In the 1920s, the work of medical education began in Switzerland and Germany and in connection with this Rudolf Steiner gave a series of lectures in 1924 which were later collected and published as the "Curative Education Course" (Steiner, 2010), or “Education for Special Needs” (2014).

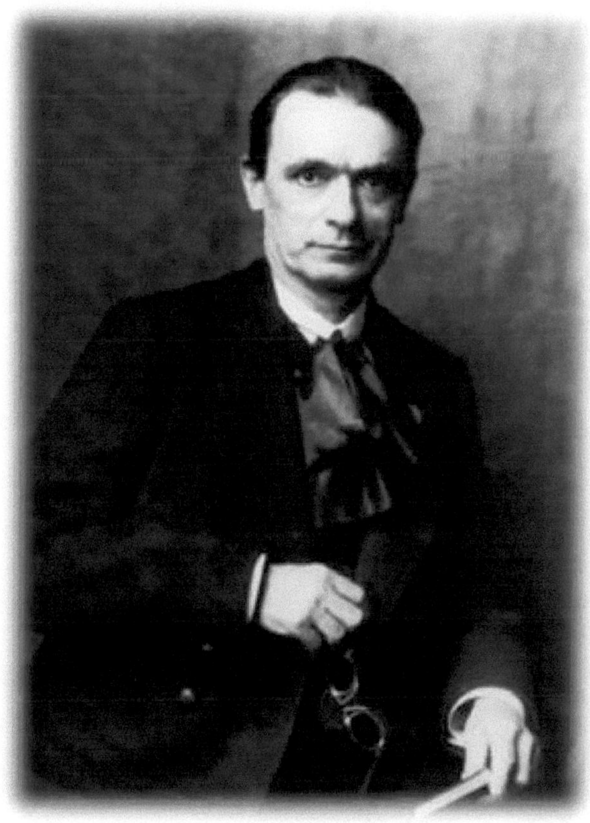

Rudolf Steiner

ANTHROPOSOPHICAL SOCIETY

The Anthroposophical Society is an organization for those who want to know anthroposophy and support the work done in many fields of life and professional areas that were inspired by anthroposophy. In seminars and conferences, in study groups and through artistic practice and opportunities are available to find out how anthroposophy can inspire new steps in life and to reveal the spiritual dimensions of existence. The Anthroposophical Society is represented in about 50 countries in the world. The Goetheanum in Switzerland is the international centre of anthroposophy for culture, research and conferences.

THE SCHOOL OF SPIRITUAL SCIENCE

The School of Spiritual Science was established in 1924 by Rudolf Steiner. As part of the school, a meditative path is described that leads to a deepened spiritual experience. This can then enrich practical as well as purely human life. To become a member of this meditative 'faculty' it is required that you are already a member of the Anthroposophical Society, and that you want to immerse yourself in anthroposophy and feel co-responsible for its tasks. As a 'Class member' you represent anthroposophy. Within the School, (or University) there are different Faculties or 'Sections'. The insights from the meditative work can inspire development in different professional areas.

DIFFERENT BRANCHES OF ACTIVITY

With anthroposophy as the starting point different ideas have arisen concerning the workings of the human being and the world. Under the umbrella of anthroposophy, the thoughts and ideas have since evolved into different practical branches of activity that can be seen as a tree with different branches coming from the same trunk or source. Here are some of the branches.

BIODYNAMIC AGRICULTURE

Biodynamic farming is a form of circular (or 'closed loop') agriculture with stricter requirements than organic agriculture. In biodynamic agriculture it is assumed that everything on the farm and in the garden forms a whole. Already in the 1920s, people began to cultivate biodynamically based on Rudolf Steiner's indications. Biodynamic vegetables are quite popular these days because they taste better than conventionally grown ones and have better nutritional value and storage capability (Demeter).

The farm is seen as a whole and should, as far as possible, be self-sufficient within the entire cycle. This means that the farmer must grow all the feed the animals need and that they, in turn, must produce the manure needed for cultivation. Biodynamic Agriculture strives for diversity, protection of the environment and natural resources.

Composting and grassland cultivation are important elements in biodynamic agriculture. 'Living soil' is necessary to get good results. This is a key concept in biodynamic farming. To obtain living soil with a lot of microorganisms, you must add organic matter and not destroy the soil with artificial fertilizers and toxins. In addition, a crop rotation system is practiced, and various preparations are used to enhance the soil.

Biodynamic agriculture and horticulture are accredited by the Demeter Association, a state-approved organization to maintain standards, cooperating with the Soil Association (organization that develops standards for organic cultivation). The farms accredited by Demeter do not use liquid manure or sludge or work in parallel with conventional cultivation. No genetically modified organisms (GMOs) may be present in or near the cultivated areas

Waldorf Education

The idea of Waldorf education is to develop the whole person based on thinking, feeling and will. The basic idea is to educate children so they can become free-thinking people who are confident and self-assured. The path to knowledge of oneself and of the world goes from the hands, through the heart and to the head as the child develops.

The lessons take place in blocks / periods in the early morning. The morning continues with theoretical topics while the afternoons are devoted to artistic and craft practice, often linked to the subject taught in the morning. Education should nourish the whole personality and should not just be a way to acquire knowledge. Different grades/classes have a different focus based on the age of the child and where the students are in their development.

The Waldorf School complies with the Education Act and the National Curriculum but also follows its own curriculum. It is "A Road to Freedom" and is based on a 12-year syllabus that will be adapted to the individual student. This means inspiring the student in a comprehensive way, practically, artistically and theoretically. Great emphasis is placed on developing independent, responsible individuals by putting emphasis on individual goals, as well as empathy and practice in social skills.

CURATIVE [THERAPEUTIC] EDUCATION

Therapeutic education is the work with children / adolescents who are disadvantaged in cognitive, emotional and social areas. The starting point is that the person's body, soul and spirit form a whole. Based on this view of the human being the entire living environment for the child /youth is consciously designed. Nutritious, biodynamic/organic and locally grown food, an aesthetically pleasing living environment are complemented by a careful structure of the day, week, month and seasons. This creates peace, security and predictability. Both curative education and therapeutic education is used. In this book are we using the word curative education from now on.

SOCIAL THERAPY

Social therapy is the work with adults who are disadvantaged in the cognitive, emotional and social areas. It has many similarities with curative education as far as the view of the holistic life situation and the design of the environment and structure, in addition to the fact that social therapy also focuses on the developmental process towards adult life and work.

ANTHROPOSOPHICAL MEDICINE

Fundamental to the anthroposophical philosophy of care is an integrative approach to health, which does not focus on a physical-biological perspective or symptoms. Elements such as closeness, touch, conversation and patience are fundamental factors. Anthroposophical medicine, mainly made from plants and minerals is given - where necessary in combination with conventional medicine - in combination with artistic therapies.

ARTISTIC THERAPIES AND OTHER THERAPEUTIC TREATMENTS

Among the artistic therapies are painting, drawing, modelling, singing and music and eurythmy. The latter is an art form originating directly from anthroposophy. It is reminiscent of dance and the movements are expressions of the soul's creative forces and energies. The eurythmist moves to the words of poetry or to music. Eurythmy is also used in pedagogy to create a visible experience of language and music. Eurythmy therapy is also available. Other therapeutic treatments include hydrotherapy, massage and 'Einreibungen', rubbing essential oil on all or parts of the body.

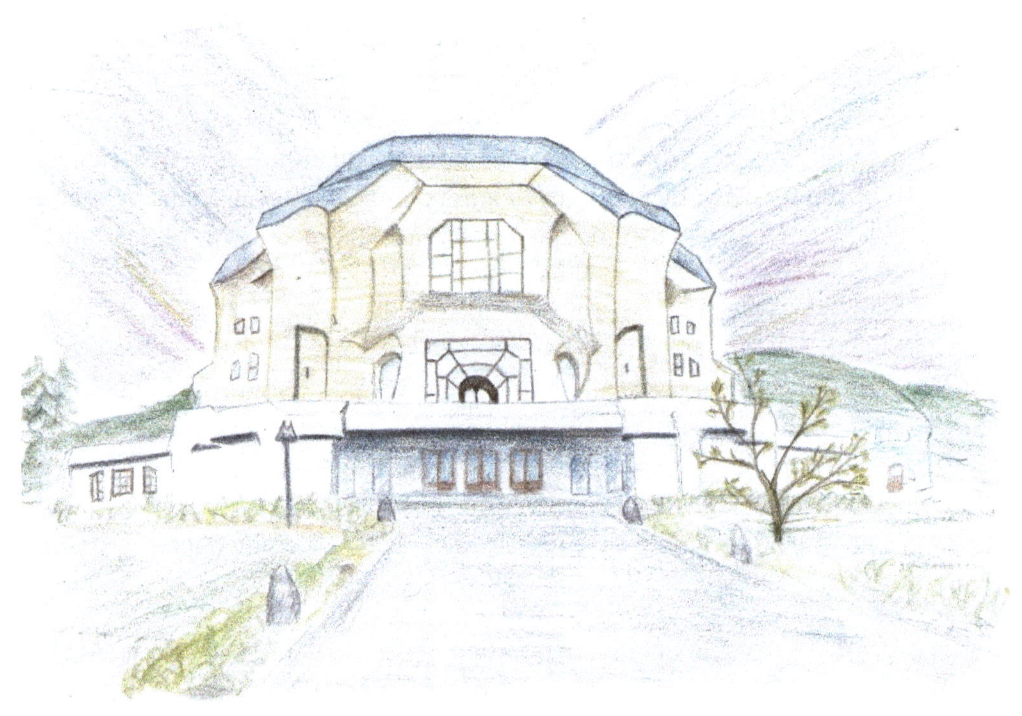

The Goetheanum

SOCIAL THERAPY - AN INTERNATIONAL MOVEMENT

Social therapy is a further development of Curative (Therapeutic) Education based on anthroposophy. 'Curative' Education was inspired by Rudolf Steiner in 1924 with the lectures of the 'Curative Education Course' and began with activities in Switzerland, Austria and Germany. The ideas spread, first within Europe but then further around the world. A focus that has been of great importance in several countries is the Camphill movement, where committed coworkers with Karl König as a front figure took the idea of curative education and began to build up centres, starting in Scotland. The whole Camphill movement began with healing education for children and young people, but in 1954 the first "village" was opened for adults with disabilities with their parents being the great driving force.

The vision from the beginning was that everyone would live in a family-like situation rather than in large dormitories and that as an adult with a disability you would be able to work in the kitchens, workshops, farm or garden on the site and thus find your place in life and in work.

There are three essentials of the Camphill organization. The first is that everyone has an "I" which is eternal and is equal regardless of disability. The person *is* not disabled, but the person *has* a disability. The second essential is that our own inner development creates the conditions for meeting the person in need of special care and support. The third essential lies in the social sphere: every person has a need for a private approach, for which opportunities for this must be created in a working community.

Today, not all institutions in Europe are part of the Camphill, but it had a great influence in the early stages, as many of the first communities were members of this movement. There are social therapeutic and curative educational communities in about 50 countries in the world, spread across all continents except in the Arctic. Everyone has their own conditions and strengths. Some organizations are small with a few people in the community, while others are large organizations with several hundred and in some cases thousands of people within their organization. In some countries there are good economic conditions with funding from the state or regions, while other places must finance themselves through fund raising, donations and sales. Many activities have initially come about through initiatives by parents or because a group of coworkers has seen a need, for instance, when school children had grown older and needed workplaces and activities adapted to adult life. Common to all is a desire to create an inclusive community where everyone can contribute their own particular strengths. Many organizations relate to national associations and regional groups. There are also several training courses and conferences in healing pedagogy and social therapy in different parts of the world, both in individual countries and through collaboration within a region.

International Anthroposophical Collaboration

The centre of anthroposophy in the world is the Goetheanum in Dornach in Switzerland. Here the School of Spiritual Science has its home. In the General 'Section' (or Faculty) of this 'High'School the anthroposophical activities are coordinated internationally. There are 11 'Sections' [Faculties] based on different areas of activity. Until now social therapy and therapeutic/curative education have been part of the Medical Section. Its subdivision, the Anthroposophic Council for Inclusive Social Development has been instrumental in forming a 12th Section, the Section for Inclusive Social Development, to be inaugurated at the October Conference 2024 in connection with the 100th anniversary of the Curative Education Course. The international work comprises a major international conference every other year and working groups on various topics, as well as annual meetings between country representatives (Delegates Meeting).

BASIC IDEAS OF ANTHROPOSOPHY AND SOCIAL THERAPY

THE POWER OF AN IDEA BRINGS ABOUT COLLEGIAL COLLABORATION

In their origin social therapy institutions share a non-profit ethos rather than an economic pursuit of profit. Organizations can be viewed from the perspective of 'social threefolding': this term is based on Rudolf Steiner's theory that organizations, as is the case in society as a whole, arise from three sub-functions which ideally need to remain in equilibrium. Resources (and distribution) form the economic basis, the legal foundations regulate social interaction, and science, education and a variety of arts shape the cultural life. The economic aspect is about ensuring that (natural) resources are managed responsibly and distributed fairly. What is produced should be in demand and then used or consumed. It is about satisfying and meeting the needs of all stakeholders. Sustainability also includes a balanced financial budget and the payment of fair wages. Regarding social and legal aspects, it is a matter of distributing relevant information, using skills, cultivating communication and showing commitment. Other important factors of well-functioning organizations are a sense of responsibility, fairness and democratic processes at all levels.

The culture of an organization includes its development and common goals, which are the driving force for all its members. Values, traditions and forms of socializing are also part of it. If several people are to work along the same lines, mission statements must be clearly defined. Managers have the task of ensuring that processes in their organization are reviewed regarding the economy, the legal situation and the culture they live in, and that decisions are made in such a way that, ideally, the three areas mutually support each other.

QUESTION FOR REFLECTION:

HOW CAN YOU CONTRIBUTE TO THE COMMUNITY/ORGANIZATION YOU ARE IN?

Based on anthroposophical values, the founders of socio-therapeutic institutions want to create living space and employment for people with disabilities. Most institutions primarily state this purpose as a corporate objective in their articles of association. If an ethos is the basis of an institution, the coworkers are of great importance as the "bearers" of this ethos.

Regarding decisions to be taken, the aim is to achieve unanimous consensus rather than mere majorities in the workforce. Of course, this cannot succeed in every case, so that sometimes decisions must be made by the management group or the person responsible for the institution. If the stakeholders understand the decisions of the management as being informed and clearly justified, good leadership can be achieved. In this way, it becomes comprehensible and transparent for the workforce and enables them to participate and collaborate.

Where groups function in this way, experienced members of staff who do not rely solely on "the management" or external prerequisites can also take on responsibility. One condition is to constantly occupy oneself with Anthroposophy including inner personal development. With their decisions, individuals support the idea of the organization and may be given great "freedom in responsibility". Staff members are potentially perceived as contributors to the success of the organization, in which all are working as equals.

The key question is: how do you create a strong organization that doesn't kill off the initiative and creativity of its staff? It is important that coworkers support the ethos and know how to make professional decisions. People come into the work with different levels of knowledge and experience. New staff members need colleagues who share their knowledge and experience.

The organization depends on coworkers who help to shape it and keep the anthroposophical idea alive with their knowledge and experience. Without this there is a risk that social therapy will dry up and become a pale copy of what it could be. At the same time, social therapy is required to be constantly developed in line with the current scientific ideas on disability, impairments and social participation.

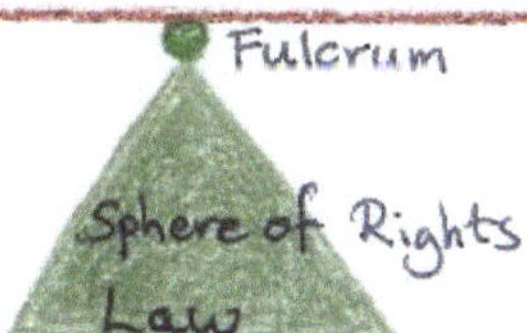

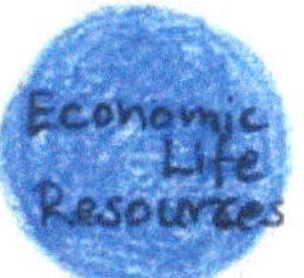

'social threefolding'

THE FOUR BODILY PRINCIPLES

From the anthroposophical viewpoint, the human being does not just have a physical body but has four bodily principles which interact with each other: physical body, ether body, astral body and self [the 'I'].

We share our physical **body** with everything in the physical world. The clearest image of a physical body could be a stone. In the stone there is no further activity apart from what it is exposed to from outside. If it rains, it gets wet and if the sun shines on the stone it dries and becomes warm.

The human **physical body** is flesh and bone and everything else that we can see and touch. It is the blood that flows around the body, intestines, tendons, fat and ultimately the skin that envelops everything. We share this bodily principle with the mineral kingdom, the plant kingdom and the animal kingdom. Matter is changeable but fixed within the physical framework. It doesn't suddenly start to grow a new arm or an ear in the middle of life. All human bodies follow a given template even though there are variations. We can objectively observe the physical: eye colour, body height, shoe size, the shape of the ear, blood pressure, the working of the metabolism.

The ether body consists of the life forces found in the physical body. Unlike stones, plants have an ether body in addition to their physical body. There is a force that makes the plant live and grow. A dehydrated plant receiving water does not only get wet, but also absorbs the water and after a while can defy gravity and begin to strive upwards again. The life processes in the plant then become stronger. The life body/ether body builds up the physical body in human beings, animals and plants.

The astral body, our soul life, we share with the animal kingdom. It works mainly in the rhythmic system as in the beating of the heart and the inhalation and exhalation of the lungs. In the astral body there are also urges, instincts, emotions such as antipathy and sympathy. Think of a thirsty dog that gets water to drink: the body becomes heavier from the water and the thirst is quenched. You could see that even before it gets the water the dog reacts because it knows that when its master or mistress picks up the bowl water will be provided. Unlike the ether body, the astral body can leave the body, for example when we sleep.

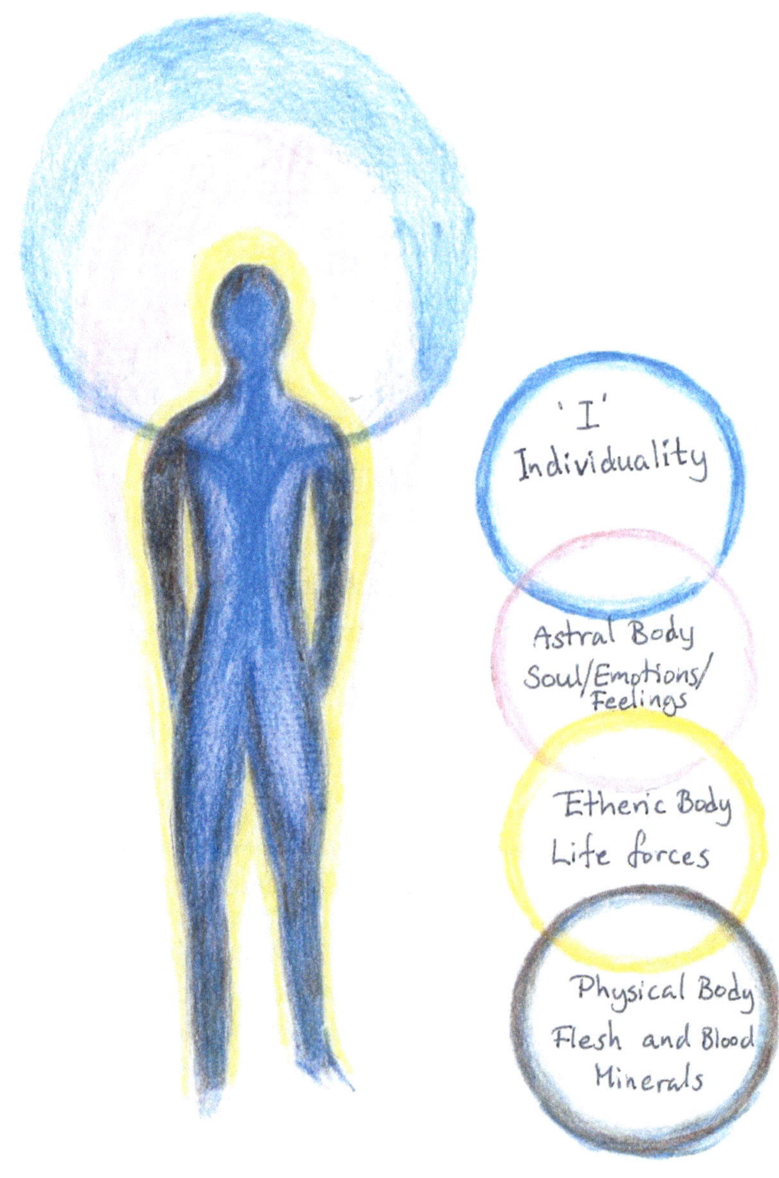

The fourfold human being as I see it.

The fourth principle is **the self/ the 'I'**, which we humans do not share with any other earthly beings. The self is our innermost core and connects the body and soul with the spiritual. With the self we can reflect on ourselves, arrive at proper judgments, develop morals and take responsibility based on freedom. A strong self can set boundaries as well as consciously break habits, compulsions and prejudices. With the self we can rein in the urges in the astral body. To return to the example of water, it can be difficult to predict what a thirsty person will do with water if access is limited. Maybe s/he drinks it all her/himself, but it can also happen that they can overcome their urge and give the water to someone else or share it. To become a skilled social therapist, one must devote a lot of time to the development of the self.

How can this be put into practice in everyday life? Among other things, this can be done by working according to the 'pedagogical law', which will be described later. This makes us aware of what needs to be strengthened in ourselves and will provide a good starting point for working on our self-development.

QUESTIONS FOR REFLECTION

TRY TO DESCRIBE YOUR PHYSICAL BODY OR THAT OF SOMEONE ELSE AS OBJECTIVELY AND IN AS MUCH DETAIL AS POSSIBLE.

HOW IS THE LIFE FORCE OF YOUR BODY? HOW IS YOUR METABOLISM, HAIR GROWTH, BODY WARMTH?

WHAT URGES DO YOU FEEL ARE STRONGEST IN YOU?

WHAT IS YOUR UNIQUE PERSONALITY?

THREEFOLDNESS

The human being from many perspectives is more than just a body. In anthroposophy one speaks of a three-fold human being. The three parts form a whole, which is larger than the sum of the parts. The different thirds, in turn, are not only interrelated, but have a connection with the four bodily principles. From this perspective, the physical body relates to the ether body, the soul to the astral body and the spirit to the 'I'. (Ritter, 2015)

THE BODY AND LIFE PROCESSES (PHYSICAL BODY)

The *Physical Body,* which is all we can see and objectively examine, is also three-fold

- **The head represents** stillness, is hard on the outside and soft inside. *Neural and sensory functions* used for thinking are in the head.

- The moveable limbs, such as **arms, legs and lower part of the trunk,** are soft on the outside and the skeleton inside is hard. Part of the metabolism takes place which is in constant motion and is as mobile as the limbs is in the trunk. These parts belong to *the metabolic and limb system***.**

- In the chest there is the *rhythmic system* of **breathing and heartbeat.** There is openness to the outside as well as in the enveloping ribs. The rhythmic system is alternately hard and soft.

- In anthroposophical medical science the threefoldness can be useful for analysing the relationship between the neural-sensory system, the rhythmical system and the metabolic-limbs system.

THE SOUL (ASTRAL BODY)

When speaking about threefoldness it is usually related to the threefold *soul,* which comprises **thinking, feelings and action.** Steiner Waldorf Education addresses all three areas equally and wants to strengthen the children in these three areas as they are growing up. Thinking, feeling and will belong together and need to be in balance. We cannot see our thoughts and feelings, they are invisible, but they are expressed in how we act and what we say and want to do.

In anthroposophy, the 'will' is something different from wishing for something or wanting to have something- as one might believe it to be- but it means doing something out of an intention; having something in mind and making it happen. A strong will allows us to manage to go against our urges, persevere and accomplish things even though they may be boring or difficult.

The Spirit ('I', the self)

The 'I', the self, can master the various processes of the body. The self is invisible but can show itself in how we think and what we do. It is active in body and soul, but can also connect with the spiritual world, independent of the physical world. When connected with the spiritual, an idea can create something new in the physical world. An openness to the spiritual allows new ideas to 'land' in us and through the body we can create something we can see and touch. The spiritual creates that which is human in the human being.

There seems to be one world of ideas, where the same idea can reach many people at the same time. In human history one can see that new inventions and hope for progress have occurred simultaneously in several people in different places of the world independent of each other.

The Wholeness

The soul and spirit need the body to express themselves. One could say that the body is the instrument, the soul plays it, and the spirit writes the music for it. Each part, in turn, is divided into three parts and these are connected to each other based on their characteristics. In the head, which is part of the body, there is thinking and stillness which in turn belong to the soul and spirit.

Our thoughts are also three-fold and can be based in the physical, the soul or the spirit depending on how we think and what we are thinking about. Just thinking about tonight's dinner and picking up the kids from preschool is quite physical. Discussing, analysing and deepening one's thoughts is connected to the soul. When we open ourselves during meditation and ruminate on the meaning of life, for example, our thoughts are on a spiritual level.

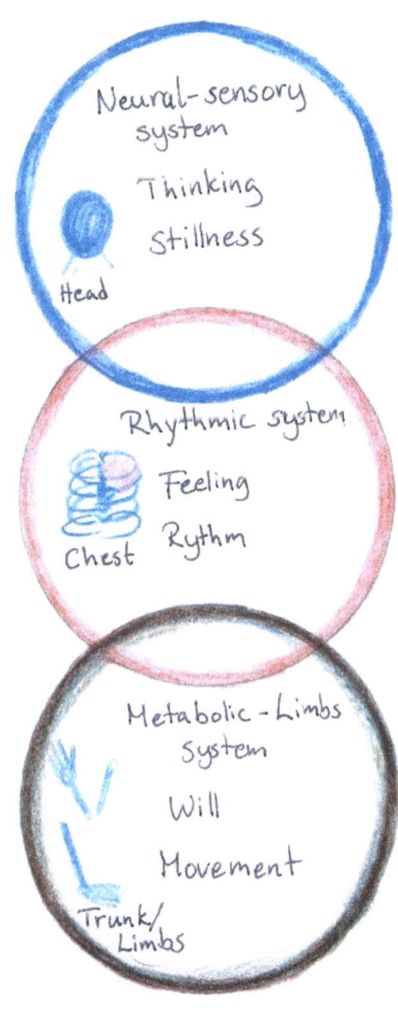

Threefoldness

How can we use this knowledge?

Thinking, feeling and action are used in Steiner Waldorf pedagogy, medical education and bringing up children, but also in social therapy and in one's self-development. Understanding how they are connected in the child's development can be helpful in finding out what you can do if there are any difficulties /disabilities during childhood. Someone who is growing up and hasn't been allowed to develop their will enough may need to practice doing more practical and artistic things as an adult. For someone who has not been able to develop their emotional life, artistic therapies but also practicing compassion and consideration for others may be needed to strengthen their morality and ethics. It is possible to strengthen thinking by practicing reasoning, analysing and discussing. We ourselves can exercise our thinking, feeling and doing by being aware of any area in which we are stronger or weaker. Everyone needs to work to develop their life of soul and spirit. You can read more about this in a short introduction on how to do this in the chapter on self-development.

It is also possible to look at illness from a three-fold perspective. We can, for instance, observe how we experience pain. In the physical body muscles and nerves might be hurting. From a soul-spiritual point of view it is all about our attitude to that which is hurting. It is possible to influence how we experience pain through our thinking. The spiritual aspect is how we relate to why we feel pain. If we can find meaning in why something is hurting, we will be able to cope with the pain on a spiritual level. (Ritter, 2015)

Questions for reflection

Are you mostly a thinking person, an emotional person or a person of action?

Can you experience how your 'I' can control your urges?

Can you become aware who leads you inwardly and who is your guide?

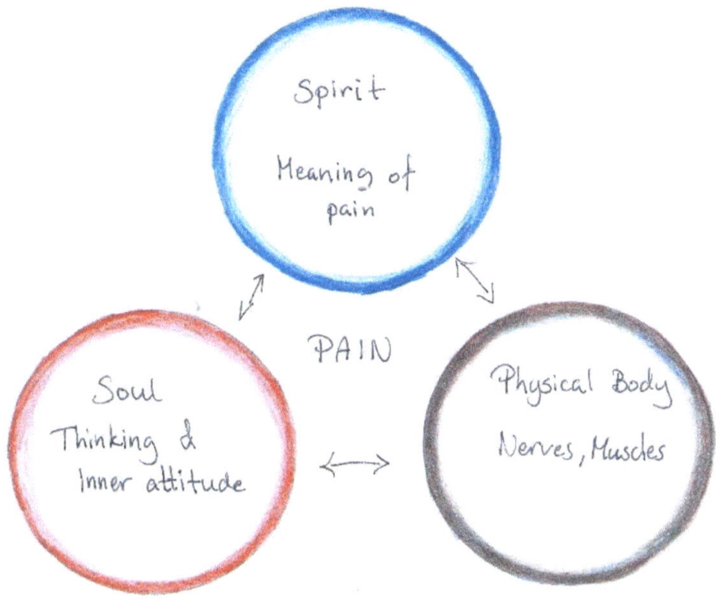

Example: Pain

THE PEDAGOGICAL LAW

We can probably all sense that other people affect us. Some make us want to act like better people, some make us feel good inside. When we are together with one person, we become brave while with another person we become cowardly and feel bad. Some seem to have it within themselves to work pedagogically or therapeutically while others simply do not despite a long training. How we influence others around us happens unconsciously to a degree. Rudolf Steiner formulated in the Curative Education Course (2010) that it is possible to see a pattern if we know what to look for. In therapeutic education we speak about the 'pedagogical law' which is based on the knowledge of the four bodily principles.

In everyday encounters we influence the person we meet through our bodily principles in different ways. When we work in a social therapeutic way or in therapeutic education, we can consciously influence the other person through our own "higher" bodily principle. This means that *the 'I' (self)* of a support worker affects the astral body of a resident / student; the astral body of a support worker affects the ether body of a resident / student, and the etheric body of a support worker affects the *physical body of a resident / student.* It is always the "higher" bodily principle that influences the one below it in the other. (Holtzapfel, 2008)

Even within our own selves the bodily principles affect each other in a downwards direction while also continually flowing "up and down". If a limb is weakened it will create a blockage which can manifest in any of the other bodily principles. For example, if we are weakened / blocked in our emotional life (the astral body) due to trauma, it may weaken our life forces. The same also applies to the forces of the 'I' and we may become more exposed to other people's emotional expressions. Physical injuries can affect our life forces which in turn affect our emotional life and mental strength. Similarly, it goes the other way too. When there is a blockage, for example, in our emotional life due to overload through stress or depression, it also affects our life forces and physical body, making us more susceptible to infections and illness. The support worker's task is to identify where there are blockages in those they support and at the same time to strengthen their own bodily principles to support the other in the best possible way.

Thus, when we use the pedagogical law, it is the higher principle in the coworker that affects the principle below it in the person being supported. It can be compared to touching your arm. The self cannot directly command the arm to move, but it goes from the self to the astral body, on to the ether body and then, finally, the arm moves in the physical body. It can be likened to the fact that the sun cannot directly shape a boulder. But through its heat, the sun can cause the water cycle to change. The water vapour rises and becomes rain which forms the water course, and which over time can grind down the stone. (Holtzapfel, 2008)

Strengthening the physical body

When the body shows various disabilities, the healthy life forces of the support worker can mitigate the symptoms. In practical terms, with genuine humour and a zest for life we can give a happy atmosphere to an experience and laugh about it heartily together. We can have a positive impact through rhythms in everyday life, clear routines, good nutritious food and warmth. (Holtzapfel, 2008). Lack of care and nursing can manifest in the physical body as delayed motor and mental development, as well as weight loss. In studies in Rumanian orphanages in the '40s, it could be seen that children separated from their mothers showed such symptoms as well as increased mortality. The children had a good chance of recovering if they were adopted or reunited with the mother within a year (Broberg et al., 2009, p 92).

Strengthening of the life forces (ether body)

Our emotional life affects those around us. If we are calm and harmonious, it rubs off on others, which manifests, among other things, in digestion, breathing, warmth and sleep. We can harness our spiritual powers by exercising objective compassion and empathy. We should not feel sorry out of mere sympathy or have antipathy but find an empathetic approach to the person we want to help. In empathy we can gain knowledge about what the other person feels and understand them on a deeper level. We can put ourselves in their situation and feel love without having the feelings they have. Through such sensitive observation a channel opens between people enabling one to feel what the other person needs. (Holtzapfel, 2008). One method of jointly finding a way to strengthen the ether body of a resident is, for example, by drawing attention to it in a staff meeting and together describing the objective conditions affecting the person who is struggling. The aim is to find a way to help them. In the collegial situation we can help each other by putting our experiences into words and sharing them with each other. Through this process, something starts to happen. On the next day what was previously a big problem may suddenly have been solved. The resident starts to act differently, and something has opened up. Especially when we meet people who have difficulty expressing themselves, we need to capture the nuances and details and through self-knowledge distinguish between that which actually happened and what was going on in our own emotional life.

Strengthening the astral body

With our 'I' we can practice reining in our own feelings in front of a person who is stuck in their emotional life so that in the situation we are not affected by the feelings of the other when they have an outburst. If we can control our thoughts, it affects our emotions and, in turn, what we do. Our attitude to and opinion of the situation has a major impact on what is happening. If we assume that the person in front of us is struggling instead of being difficult, we enhance the effect we have. If we go in with the conviction that it will work, the chances of it doing so also increase. Another way to support our thinking is to think carefully and create action plans for different situations. Then we are inwardly strengthened and by being mentally present we spread security around us, which supports those who do not manage their own emotions and their astrality very well. Sensitive people feel our presence, which gives them security. When we are not present mentally or distracted by other thoughts, it creates a void which produces a feeling of chaos within the person. (Holtzapfel, 2008)

Knowing more about the person we are going to help will make our 'I' more secure so we will be mentally more stable in the situation. If I as a support worker know and understand why something is the way it is, I will be able to accept the person more easily and become more involved with them. My 'I' can also be strengthened if a conversation with someone else makes us change our mind about a situation. In this way we can meet a person who is overcome by their emotions with more clarity. If we can consciously realize that the other person's feelings are not about us, we also find it easier to create a certain distance from the feeling. We can work preventively by stimulating the imagination of the other, for example by making up stories together, fantasizing together and playing.

Strengthening the self

If we must strengthen someone else's powers of the 'I', we need the help of our higher selves. In concrete terms, the support worker can strengthen the individual's self by speaking in different ways, for instance by being over-explicit in enunciating or maybe even exaggerating it. Practicing eurythmy and storytelling are good tools to use. Moral stories such as folktales also strengthen the self by showing in narrative form what is morally right and wrong. Our own selves can be strengthened through regular meditation so that we can get in touch with our higher selves. (Holtzapfel, 2008)

Skilled social therapists / therapeutic educators strive to identify where in the different bodily principles there are blockages in the person in front of them, so they will be able to use themselves as a tool to influence and help. We need to develop our intuition by continuing to develop ourselves consciously so we can find out the right thing to do for each individual person. The way we work with ourselves and support each other affects our way of working and its success.

QUESTIONS FOR REFLECTION

CAN YOU IDENTIFY ANY OBVIOUS BLOCKAGE IN ANY BODILY PRINCIPLE IN YOURSELF?

CAN YOU IDENTIFY ANY BLOCKAGE IN A PERSON IN YOUR SURROUNDING?

CAN YOU THINK BACK TO A SITUATION IN WHICH BY WORKING ON YOURSELF YOU WERE ABLE TO CHANGE A SITUATION?

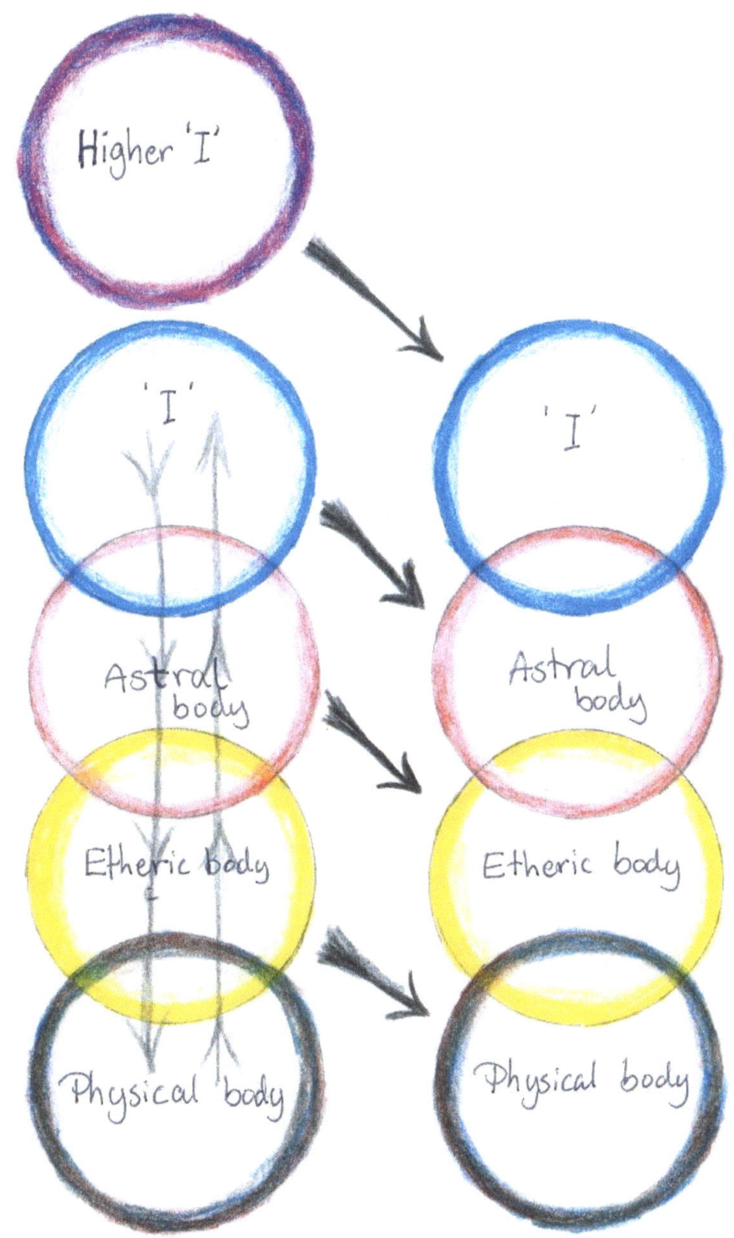

The law of education as it may operate within us and vis-à-vis others.

THE FOUR TEMPERAMENTS

Four children are walking on a path through the forest. Suddenly, there is a fallen tree on the path. The first child is skipping with light steps along the path, almost as if it is hovering a little above the ground while moving its feet lightly. When the child arrives at the tree it takes a single leap and continues skipping, almost as if it didn't notice that there was something in the way. This is the 'sanguine' person.

The second child is walking on the path with firm steps. It walks on with confidence and a vigorous spring in the step. Arriving at the tree, the child picks up a thick branch and tries to pull the tree away from the path, slaving away and working hard until the sweat is running down. When the tree does not move, the child gets angry and kicks at it. This is the 'choleric' person.

Child number three is walking along the path with a dreamy gaze. It looks at the flowers in the grass and listens to the chirping of the birds. The child may have a sweet bun in its backpack for the picnic, for it is important not to go hungry. Arriving at the tree trunk, it stands there for a while to think and then walks leisurely around the crown of the tree and continues the journey. This is the 'phlegmatic' person.

The last child is walking with heavy steps, immersed in thoughts. The body is gangly and slightly bent over as if the body does not quite fit. When the child arrives at the tree, it sinks down on the trunk and sighs to itself. " Typical that there should be a tree right there where *I'm* going to go. It's always going to happen to *me*." This is the 'melancholic' person.

The different children characterize the four temperaments which mark us out. In each child one temperament is more prominent and it can be seen by the child's appearance which temperament is the strongest. In adults, one temperament is more prominent but is complemented by a second one which can also be seen clearly. The four temperaments are strongly connected to the four bodily principles and reflected in the physical body (Steiner, 1999)

The sanguine person is sociable and easy-going, not burdened by problems but rather unaware of them. At the party, the sanguine person is the one who mingles and talks to everyone. On the other hand, there may not be long serious conversations with them.

They are the one in a group who has ideas and gets people going, invents wonderful new projects but is not very good at keeping them up and thinking them through to the end.

The energetic choleric person wants to get into action, overcome problems and fight hard. They do not give up easily after the first attempt. Around a choleric, things happen, often in a forceful way. In the heat of battle the choleric does not give in. Confrontations easily happen if others disagree.

The phlegmatic takes most things with equanimity. They can work on seemingly boring tasks for long periods of time and have the patience to keep going on and on. However, they can become a little too dreamy at times and sudden changes are not welcomed. There is not much that gets a phlegmatic person off balance, though they may need to be woken up occasionally.

The melancholic person lives in their own mind, pondering and analyzing, is sometimes a little over the top and downcast. They can go deeply into things and a melancholic person can also really listen to other people.

Knowing the temperaments can give us a better understanding of how a person 'ticks' and what is easy or difficult for them. It is also exciting to be aware of one's own temperaments so we can work towards an increased balance between our different temperaments and characteristics.

QUESTIONS FOR REFLECTION

WHICH MAIN TEMPERAMENT(S) DO YOU RECOGNIZE IN YOURSELF?

CAN YOU IDENTIFY PEOPLE AROUND YOU WHO HAVE STRONG TRAITS OF A PARTICULAR TEMPERAMENT? WHICH ONE?

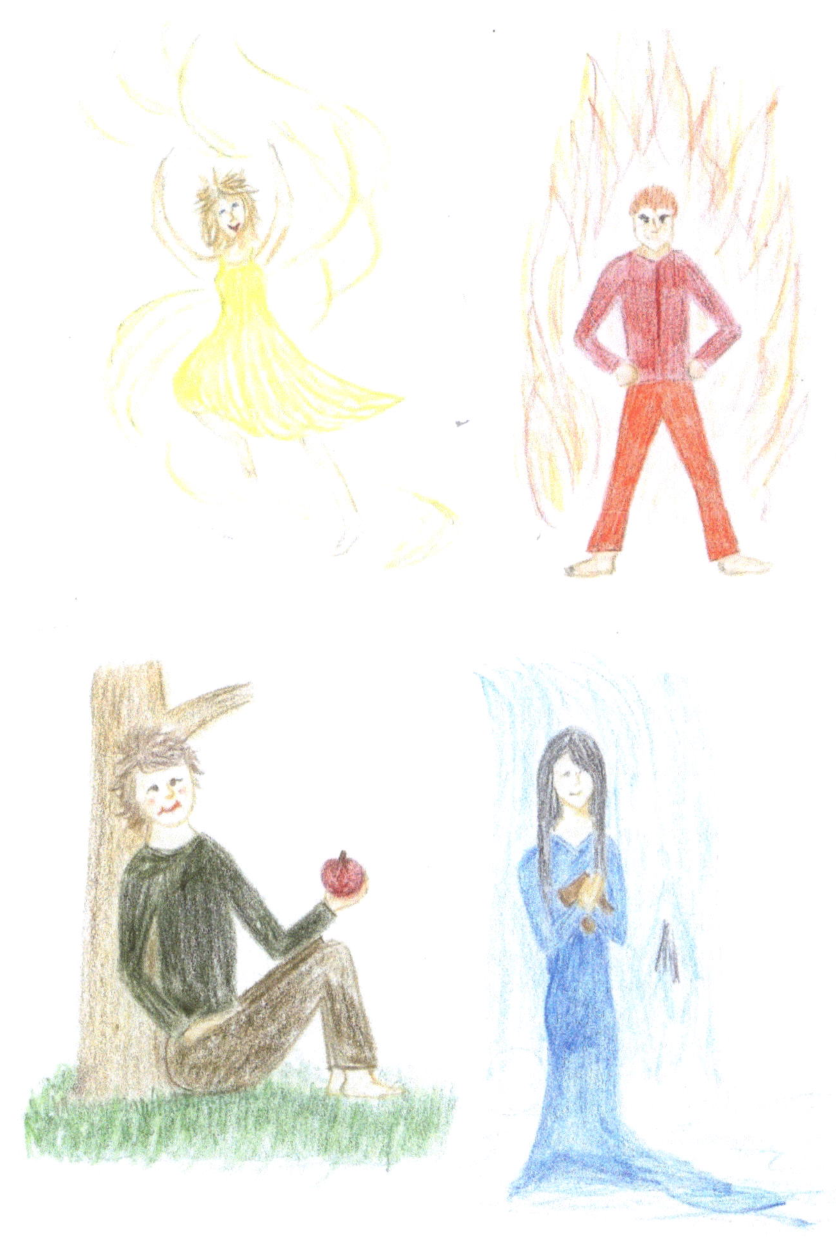

The four children with different temperaments as one can imagine them to look like.

POINT AND CIRCLE

In the Curative Education Course (2010), Rudolf Steiner addressed the polarity of 'point and circle', which is, simply speaking, about concentration/ contraction into a point and widening/ expansion into a circle. Imagine a point centering into its most concentrated form until it is no longer visible or measurable. If the point cannot be concentrated any further, the movement will continue within itself and begin to expand again. The same is true for the circle, in that it expands indefinitely until the circumference of the circle is so large that it becomes straight. If the movement continues, the direction begins to change. The interior of the circle now becomes its exterior and vice versa.

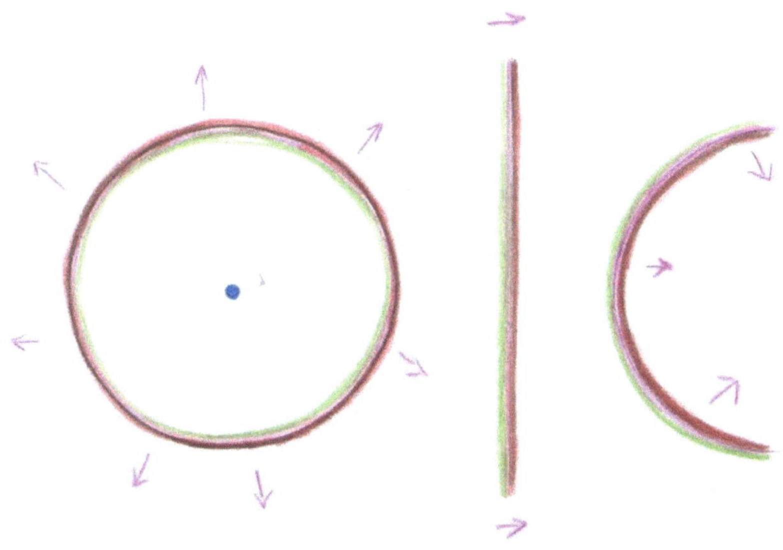

The circle continues outward until it changes direction

In social therapy and therapeutic education, we consciously work with the fact that we as human beings have 'point' or 'circle' tendencies within us. Some people hang on tightly to the point while becoming introverted and cramped up, while others flow out into the surroundings and find it difficult to set boundaries for themselves. One can see that human beings tend to go more in one or the other direction, which is more and less outspoken depending on the time of day. In the morning, we are more focused, awake and receptive to the outside world (point tendencies), while in the evening we are more open and dissipated (circle tendencies). If it goes too far in any direction, it becomes an unhealthy one-sidedness. Getting caught up in obsession is the extreme form of the point tendency while hypersensitivity and worry/anxiety are the circle tendency.

In the healthy state, there is a constant interchange between the extreme forms. Sometimes one can get stuck in one extreme and then help is needed to free oneself from it and get back into the rhythm. The goal is not to strive for the opposite but move rhythmically between the polarities. Think of it as a pendulum movement which should swing out ever more widely. The understanding of the importance of rhythm can also be used in relation to sleep - the higher the degree of wakefulness you can achieve in the morning, the easier it is to get to sleep in the evening.

Point tendencies	**Circle tendencies**
Memory	Forgetfulness
Waking up	Falling asleep
Stillness	Movement

QUESTIONS FOR REFLECTION

FIND OUT IF YOU CAN NOTICE IN YOURSELF ANY DIFFERENCE BETWEEN MORNING AND EVENING

DO YOU HAVE MORE 'POINT' TENDENCIES OR 'CIRCLE' TENDENCIES IN YOURSELF?

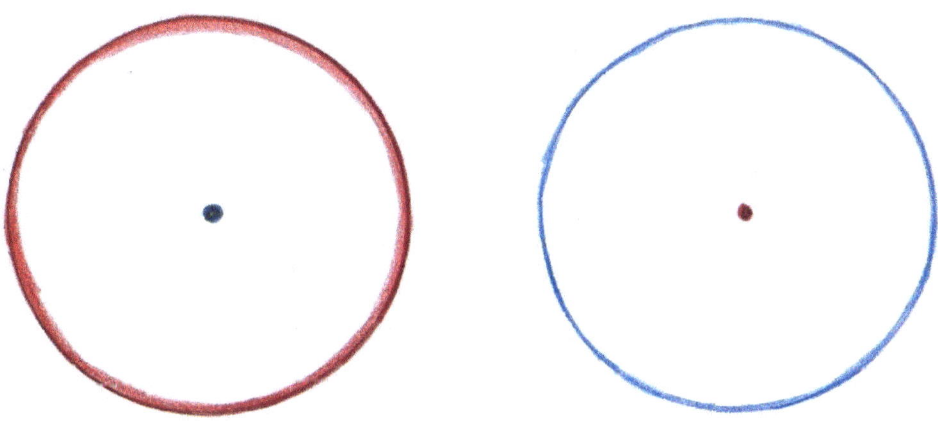

Circle and point/point and circle

POLARITIES OF HUMAN CONSTITUTIONAL TYPES

The concept of point and circle is also helpful for characterizing or understanding the other polarities described by Steiner in the Curative (Therapeutic) Education Course. Steiner describes a polarity such as "hysteria" or "epilepsy". The "hysteric" tendency is more circular, going towards the outside, while the "epileptic" tendency is more point-like, going inwards. We are all inclined to either one or the other. No human being is in perfect balance, yet if it deviates too far in one direction, it becomes problematic.

Being aware of one's own constitution or that of those around you helps in understanding people's behaviour or how they interact with their surroundings.

To put it simply, a "hysterical" person has a filter that is too permeable and lets in too much of the environment. That of the "epileptic", on the other hand, lets in too little. Through various artistic therapies, the therapist can help to harmonize the one-sidedness to get closer to the middle. But this must be practiced a lot.

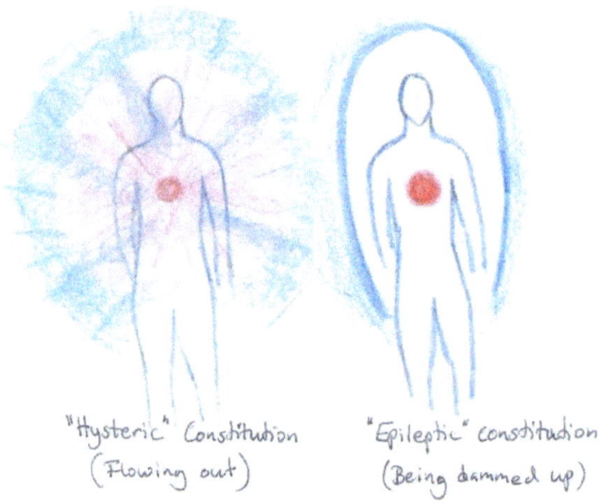

Hysteric and epileptic constitutions

Having a hysterical constitution is like sitting in a sieve to seek protection. This does not give enough protection by any means, as everything flows through it. The skin feels too thin, too sensitive, you are almost skinless. All the feelings you perceive in people around you flow straight into you as through a sieve. Things "getting under your skin" is a phrase that describes people with a hysterical tendency. They are sensitive and their vulnerability to the feelings of others allows them to "read" their surroundings well. A person with a hysterical tendency feels moods and feelings and can hardly switch them off. In connection with such a constitution, eczema and other skin problems are quite common. It is important to take people with this tendency seriously and to help them control their emotions. Change frightens them, which is why it is good to introduce it to them step by step and in a way appropriate for them.

Having a constitution termed "epileptic" feels emotionally like being locked up in a totally dark room or in a glass globe. It is hard to read other people's feelings or find out what you feel inside yourself and convey that to others. An outside observer may assume that people with epilepsy are insensitive and have no feelings, but it is really an inability to communicate one's feelings or to recognize feelings in others. This may be due to tension building up within themselves, which is discharged in epileptic seizures. This is followed by a period of relaxation. Sudden changes can sometimes help to release the tension. A good fit of laughter or emotional outburst also has a cathartic effect. People with an epileptic constitution can focus very well and usually have no problem with changes. An epileptic constitution does not necessarily mean having epileptic seizures of any kind, but rather means having a constitutional tendency. Today, Steiner's designations of curative educational illnesses (epileptic - hysterical) are replaced by descriptive terms such as congested/introverted/closed" or "flowing out/extroverted/losing oneself" (Martin Niemeijer, 2004).

Questions for Reflection

Are you more in the direction of hysteria or of epilepsy as described in the Curative Education Course?

Do you know someone with extreme epileptic traits?

Can you think of a person with strong hysteric traits?

THE TWELVE SENSES

The senses of sight, hearing, taste, smell and touch are the ones we are most familiar with, but Rudolf Steiner found in his research that the human being has twelve senses and that they form a whole. None of these senses operate independently but are connected in various ways. Based on what our senses convey to us, we create a picture of the world around us. (Wilmar, 2008).

The twelve senses can be divided into three parts:

- The sense of hearing, the sense of *word, the sense of thought and the sense* of ego (self) turn towards the outside world (thinking).
- Through the sense of smell, the sense of taste, the *sense of sight and the sense of warmth,* one meets oneself in the outer world (feeling).
- The sense of touch, the *sense of life, the sense of self-movement and the sense of equilibrium* form a group that perceives one's own body (the will).

The senses can also be seen in polarities in that one sense might work together with another one to develop itself.

The sense of touch spreads throughout the skin and is situated in thin nerve fibers underneath the outermost layer of skin. An experience of touch is turned inward. The sense of touch interacts with the sense of equilibrium to tell us whether we are sitting, standing or lying down. The sense of touch gives one the experience of one's own self. Therefore, we 'pinch ourselves' when we experience something out of the ordinary to get the feeling that I am the one experiencing this.

The sense of life is linked to the general feeling of well-being or discomfort and the whole range in between. With this mind, we experience hunger, difficulty in breathing, fatigue and general lethargy. The degree to which we are aware of the sense of life varies. It gives us a sense of existence.

The sense of (self-)movement can make us aware that we are moving. It can be trained by practicing artistic forms of expression. A harmonious sense of self-movement allows us to move without apparent effort. If this sense does not function, we become clumsy, stiff, and perhaps paralysed.

The sense of equilibrium allows us to sense the position of our body in relation to the horizontal. If we have a fall or ride a roller-coaster, we become extra aware of our sense of equilibrium. Disturbances in the sense of balance can cause dizziness and be perceived as very disturbing. A clear example of this is when we get seasick and we feel that our balance is disturbed.

The sense of smell in human beings is quite primitive organically, but despite this, we can distinguish the different scents around us. Smells can call up emotions and memories which were deep down in our consciousness. The sense of smell puts us in touch with the surrounding world.

The sense of taste is located in the mouth, in the mucous membranes and on the tongue. It is strongly linked to the sense of smell. With an unspoilt sense of taste, we are able to sense what is good or bad for our health and what our body needs. Artificial sweeteners and chemical taste enhancers can interfere with the sense of taste, for example too many sweets at an early age. (Wilmar, 2008)

The sense of sight that is situated in the eyes is a mobile sensory organ. It gives us a three-dimensional experience of the world around us, of colour and shape, distance and relationship between things. We do not only see colours but also experience opposite colours. For instance, if we look at an object for a long time and then look at a white wall, we see its complementary colours.

The sense of warmth helps us sense our own temperature and the temperature in the air and of things around us. In relation to our own temperature, we can experience whether something is hot or cold. The sense of warmth belongs to the group of emotionally related senses.

The sense of hearing, through the way it has been formed, can capture oscillations and vibrations through the air. Noise, sounds, tones and speech sounds can be captured by hearing. By consciously listening or not listening we can regulate hearing. Human beings can also create harmonious sounds that are perceived musically.

The sense of word allows us to distinguish speech from a cacophony of other sounds. Hearing alone does not provide a sense of language. Already early on in their development children begin to form speech sounds and to understand language. Culture is created through language. It allows us to capture and convey soul and spiritual contents to our fellow human beings. The sense of word is related to our power of forming pictures and ideas.

The sense of thought or concept allows us to read other people's thoughts with the help of all our senses. We get an impression of what others are thinking through what they say, through facial expressions and body language. Our concepts help us understand ourselves as well as ourselves in relation to others.

The sense of ego (self) which radiates from the head into the body makes it possible to perceive and understand our own self and that of others. Through it, we can make efforts to experience ourselves and who we are in relation to others. (Wilmar, 2008)

QUESTIONS FOR REFLECTION

WHILE SITTING DOWN AND OBSERVING YOURSELF, WHICH SENSE IMPRESSIONS CAN YOU BECOME AWARE OF?

DO YOU NOTICE ANY DIFFERENCE IF IT IS QUIET AND CALM AROUND YOU OR LOUD AND LIVELY?

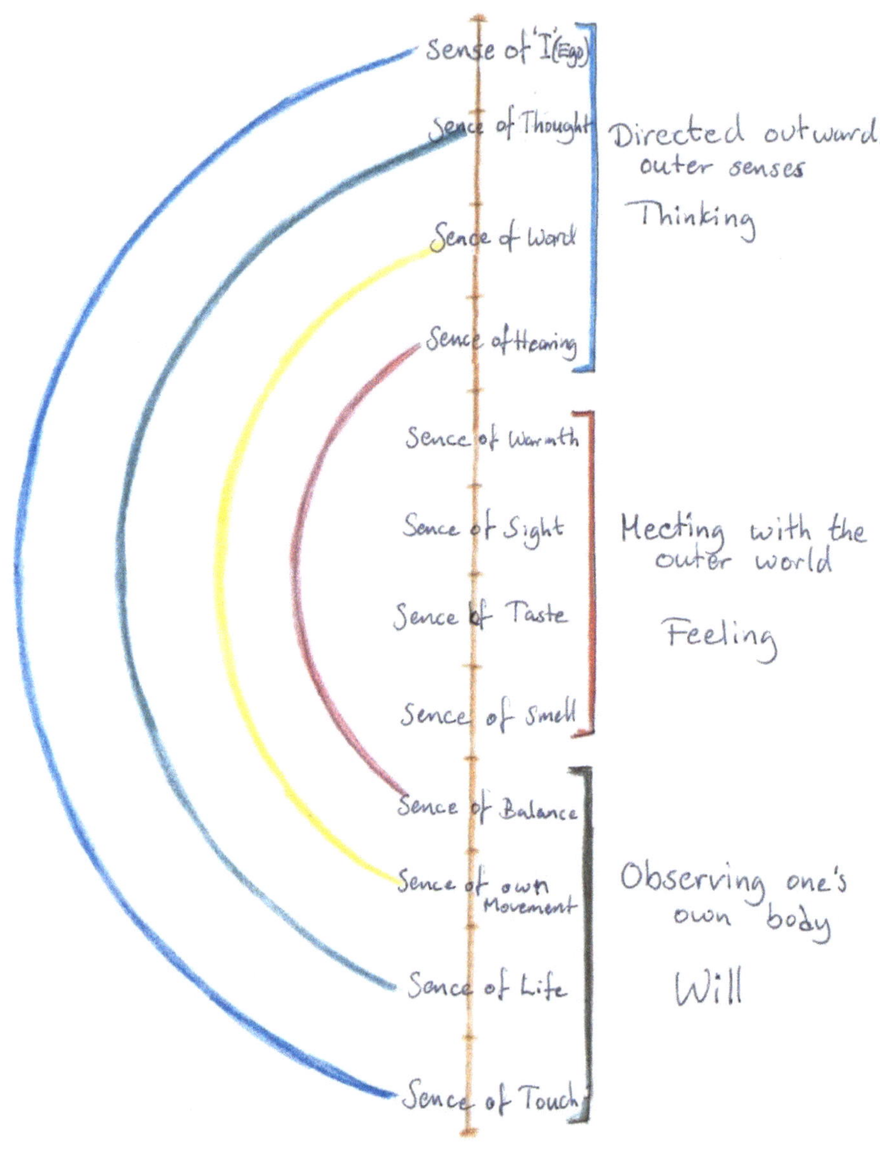

The senses and how they relate to each other.

REINCARNATION AND KARMA

In Anthroposophy, reincarnation is seen as a fact, which means that the 'I' is reborn again and again. Death is not the end, but life continues in another dimension in the spiritual world. The 'I' processes the life we have lived and traces the direction for the life to come. We can assume that we are not human beings with spiritual experiences, but spiritual beings with human experiences. The anthroposophical path of inner training gives one the opportunity to consciously connect with the spiritual world. The idea of reincarnation applies not only to every single individual, but also comprehensively to humanity around the world, which evolves in cycles.

To work in a social therapeutic organization, you don't have to believe in reincarnation, but believing that it is possible can help. One might be a bit humble when meeting another person and think to yourself: 'in another life I could be in their situation'. If taking the idea of karma as a starting point, it might well make higher sense that the two of us meet. Broadly speaking, the idea of reincarnation assumes that our soul and spirit - before being born on earth - decide on the intention they want to pursue in their coming life. Might it be to develop certain qualities? To meet certain people to bring this about? So, before my birth I have an idea of what I want to achieve in this life and which important people will have a greater influence on my personal karma. In a way it is like an inkling of my karma. Then, when we are born, we don't remember it any longer. But the people we encounter and the challenges we come across guide us if we are open to them. Life on earth has meaning because we can have experiences in the physical body and thus develop (new) qualities. From this basis, however, we always have free choice in every situation as to how we deal with what is happening around us. Decisions we make in life also influence what happens to us in the future. Crises we get into can be a powerful tool for our karma to make us see what we need to change or learn.

Due to the rebirth that takes place again and again, our fate is not only tied to the people we currently meet, but connections are also formed on a higher level. We meet people from whom we are supposed to learn something, and others meet us so that they can learn from us. It's not about factual knowledge, but about acquiring self-knowledge. For instance, we meet a person who annoys us. Perhaps we need to learn to accept the otherness of different people or to protect our own integrity from them. Karma can also mean that we get into situations that are difficult for us. Maybe they happen so we can learn to deal with difficulties or make decisions in a different way, in order not to have to face the problem again in the future.

BIOGRAPHY

Our lives can be seen in periods of seven years, each of which has a certain direction and follows certain inner laws. It is not really the case that on our birthday something completely new happens, but for some the transition to the next period occurs a little earlier and for others a little later. In addition to the seven-year periods, there are occasions in life called lunar nodes related to the course of the moon through the constellations. These occur approximately at 18.5 years, 37 years and 56 years of age. At these times in life, we may come to new insights if we are open to them. At about the age of 18 we can discover what we want to do in our lives. (Ritter, 2006)

By looking back at our life, we can learn something about ourselves. We can look at what we remember and think about why we remember a particular event. We can also see if there are certain laws in life which explain why something is happening. Are there people who have had a great impact on my life? Which encounters have influenced the choices I have made in life? Looking back at your biography will differ from time to time according to where you are in life.

Biography can be made visible by entering important events as biographical curves in the diagram as pictured below. Then we may be able to see recurring patterns, events that stand out, or turning points.

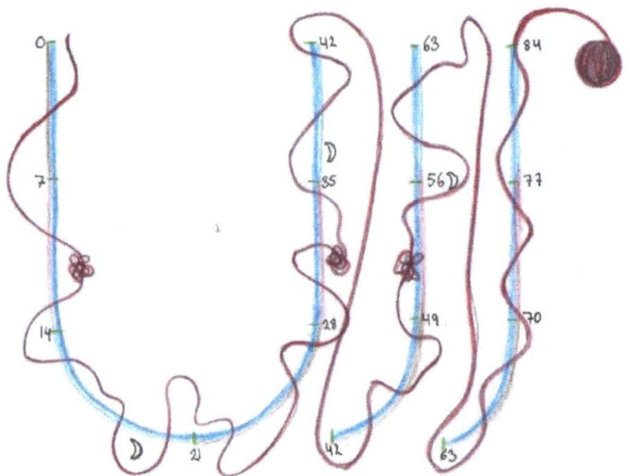

Biography arcs show how the "red thread" runs through life, how it sometimes gets tangled and how it continues on.

THE SEVEN-YEAR PERIODS
0-21 YEARS

0-7: PERIOD OF WILL AND A NEW BEGINNING – DEVELOPING THE BODY AND MOTOR SKILLS

The first seven years lay the foundation for our physical body but also a foundation for our relationship with others. An inner security can be built up in relation to the immediate family. At the age of three the child begins to be able to look at himself as an individual and to say: "I want to". The development of the brain is very important in this phase, and it would ideally allow the creation of one's own imagination and inner images without already being intellectually overburdened. In the development of the life of will, it is more important what we as educators and supporting adults do than what we say. Neither the thinking nor the emotional life is developed enough to be able to make assessments or judgments.

7-14: PERIOD OF RHYTHM, HARMONIZATION AND BALANCE

This period is characterized by the development of creativity and emotional life. The foundation has now been laid to be able to start school and the child gradually begins to form its own relationships outside the family. School (esp. Waldorf education) focuses on acquiring knowledge through experience and stories, and on expressing creativity through writing, drawing and storytelling. Emotional life continues to develop and connects learning to artistic activities and rhythms. The child learns through stories, pictures, movement and trying things out in practice.

14-21: PUBERTY AND ADOLESCENCE, DISSOLVING AND QUESTIONING - STRONG EMOTIONS

The child leaves childhood and enters adolescence. Intellectual thinking skills are being developed and honed. The body changes with puberty and the brain makes developmental leaps. One becomes mature and continues to mature to face the outside world and take responsibility. Now young people are developing their own life of thought. This makes it possible for them also to learn through their intellect. Speeding up development too much and starting with a lot of intellectualizations too early does not give a positive result in the long run.

21-42 YEARS

21-28: GETTING TO GRIPS WITH THE BASICS OF LIFE - APPRENTICE YEARS, 'GAP YEAR'

This is a time of exploring the world and wandering out into life. It is still a time of adolescence and a time to free oneself from one's childhood to find one's own path and approach. We are becoming more and more skilled in dealing with our stormy emotional life although our own feelings still have a strong grip on us.

28-35: BRINGING ORDER AND BUILDING A CAREER, ESTABLISHING AND ORGANIZING ONESELF

Occasional introspection makes us more aware of our actions and we act more consciously and purposefully. Career, family, work and private life are central in life, and it is becoming important to create a stable and secure life.

35-42: A SECOND PUBERTY – REORIENTATION REGARDING THE COMPLETION OF DUTIES.

Now we are in the middle of life and perhaps at the peak of our career, and we begin to question some of our values and goals. We search for deeper values and a lasting meaning to life. Many people are experiencing a kind of life crisis at this age. We might discover a direction in which we can find the meaning of life again in our soul and spirit.

42-63 YEARS

42-49: CREATIVITY AND BRINGING FORM, SPIRITUAL DEVELOPMENT

Broadened perspectives, a fresh start and spiritual orientation. Going more into depth, or finding a new direction is central in this phase. Spiritual maturity may be achieved if we are open to working on ourselves. Many people feel the need for new order and emancipation. It is like a new 'puberty', with the risk that it is an escape from one's own life situation and being led into emptiness. A fresh start is needed, and a new direction will come if we dare to listen inwardly and are open to what comes towards us.

49-56: Distance, Wisdom and Insight

In this phase of life, which is characterized by deceleration and stabilization, there is a need to stop and look back and reflect on the life lived so far. Many people experience an inner peace.

56-63: Seriousness and Overview

Now the retirement age is gradually approaching and with it the insight that this life is not eternal. A sense of urgency and not wanting to waste time may arise. The forces of the body are not as strong any longer and the life forces begin to withdraw. How do we deal with this? If we direct ourselves to external factors such as physical fitness, it may be more difficult to cope with it. Enriching our life with spirituality, however, will give us strength to find the way towards something new.

63-84 Years

63-70: A New Freedom

Retirement starts for most people. We might find a new meaning in everyday life or feel an emptiness without work to do. We can have more time for cultural and spiritual development. For some people, not being professionally occupied can turn into a crisis. For others it is like a new adolescence which is making it possible to explore the world.

70-77: Inner Contemplation and Becoming

The body no longer functions the way we would like it to. Breaks are becoming more and more important. Perhaps we can develop respect for the life we have lived and find some kind of peace with it.

77-84: With Death as a Companion – A Time of Saying Goodbye. One's Soul and Consciousness are Gradually Freeing Themselves from the Physical Body

The older we get, the more we withdraw into ourselves. Perhaps we are reevaluating our views of the world. The surroundings become less interesting. The soul is gradually freeing itself from the body and preparing to leave earthly life. If you live after 84, everything does not end suddenly but continues in the direction we are heading in already.

BIOGRAPHY AS A SOCIAL THERAPEUTIC TOOL

The social therapist can make visible the common thread in a person's life by researching and writing down the person's biography. The support staff team familiarizes itself with it and updates it every few years. The social therapist can also help people with disabilities to see their own common thread and gain an understanding of their own life. If possible, people in need of support will be helped to find their own red thread in their lives, thus finding an ever better understanding of their own biography. Useful ways to do this are, for instance, to collect pictures, create a photo album or make a record of a journey. A red thread can become visible through talking with each other about things that happened and remembering them together.

Finding out about another person's biography is in social therapy a way to learn to understand a person with a disability in more depth. We can find out what the person has been through in life so far and whether any major life events have taken place. From this we gain a greater understanding of certain forms of behaviour as well as insight into the fact that certain things have influenced the person’s life.

People follow similar patterns in their biographical development, but if you have an intellectual disability, there may be several parallel developments taking place. On the one hand there is the mental age with its related intellectual skills, and the biological age on the other hand. These can be quite different from each other. If there are no clear external factors, a sudden change in behaviour may be related to the person moving into the next seven-year period or into a moon node. (Ritter, 2006)

QUESTIONS FOR REFLECTION

CAN I SEE A CERTAIN PATTERN IN MY LIFE?

DO I ALWAYS END UP IN THE SAME TYPE OF CONFLICTS/DIFFICULTIES?

HAVE I EXPERIENCED UNEXPECTED LIFE-CHANGING EVENTS?

WHICH PEOPLE HAVE BEEN INSTRUMENTAL IN WHAT I HAVE DONE IN MY LIFE?

CAN I FIND OR CREATE A RECORD OF THE BIOGRAPHY OF THE PEOPLE I WORK WITH?

SELF-DEVELOPMENT/INNER PATH

Firstly, do we really need to develop? Depending on what we believe in and strive for, we may answer this question a little differently. In anthroposophy, self-development is an obvious responsibility we have as human beings. We can consciously change both physically, in soul and in spirit. Body, soul and spirit are all interconnected, and each affects the others. If the soul develops, this will also influence the body and the spirit. Self-development is aimed at discovering, consciously developing and bringing equilibrium into one's inner nature. In this way a balance is created between being open to the demands of the external world and developing inner strength and endurance.

We do not only need to work for our physical health through exercise, training and diet, but also to focus on our mental development and well-being. The soul and spirit need nourishment and development, and they can be stimulated through literature, art, meaningful conversation and reflection.

It takes some effort to bring this about. Change will happen in our lives whether we like it or not. Life gives us the opportunity to develop by providing us with all kinds of difficulties. Sometimes we are helped by external factors such as crises or events in our lives that force us to change. But we ourselves also need to take responsibility for further development. If we really want to understand something, it will be easier to do so if we put aside egotism and physical needs and act like a true human being.

Many anthroposophical texts can feel hard and difficult to read. Anthroposophical texts can touch the human being on a deeper level if one does not only read them in an intellectual way but also experiences what one reads. A wise person once said: "right now I may not be ready for this particular text". The same text may be completely obvious a few years later and you cannot trace back why you did not manage to understand it before. Often you may only understand a text when the content is relevant in your private or professional life.

Everyone should have the opportunity to develop throughout their lives, regardless of the energy a person may need for it. Therefore, we as social therapists need to think about how we can help those we support to develop and have opportunities to learn new things throughout life.

We do not only develop individually 'in our little room' for ourselves. A larger group can also be useful for creating a space for reflection or to create distance from a situation. This can be done by starting staff meetings with studying a text together and discussing the content afterwards. Then we can gain a distance from everyday problems and turn to more fundamental life issues. The more daily tasks you must accomplish, the more important it is to spend time studying together with colleagues. You then lay a common ground as a group and can then be strengthened in addressing everyday problems and issues. A study does not always have to be theoretical but could also be done in an artistic or therapeutic way such as jointly meditating, singing, practicing eurythmy etc.

QUESTIONS FOR REFLECTION

HOW DOES MY OWN INNER DEVELOPMENT RELATE TO EXTERNAL DEVELOPMENT?

WHAT DO I NEED TO DEVELOP/TRAIN IN MYSELF?

MEDITATION AND PRACTICE

One way to work on your self-development and to strengthen your (higher) self is to practice meditation. Meditation aims to develop inner sensory organs/ 'soul eyes' which can perceive phenomena in a soul and spiritual world free from the physical world - a world of imagination, inspiration and intuition. They connect the spiritual within the human being with the spiritual world. There are several different ways to meditate as well as other exercises to strengthen oneself.

Rudolf Steiner developed short exercises that can be practiced daily to work on the ability to control *thinking*, *will and feeling*, *to be positive, open-minded* and to find an *inner balance between these qualities*. (Steiner, 2019)

In a meditation to develop mobility in thinking one concentrates on an object or symbol. One could also read a verse daily, such as the weekly verses of Rudolf Steiner's *Calendar of the Soul* and ponder about it. Other exercises may include doing a review of the day before going to sleep. The review is done backwards and covers the day's events and the people we have encountered. The idea is not to fall back into how we felt at the time of our experience, but to look at the events objectively.

As a meditative exercise we could change the fixed location of an object. Put your toothbrush in a different place from usual and see how long it takes until you automatically reach for the toothbrush in its new place. When that happens, it is time to change the place again. In this way, we strengthen our will.

Another concentration exercise is to take an everyday object such as a shell, a match or a stone and sit with it in your hand and observe the object for about five minutes every day; this is a way of observing objectively. When we observe something for a long time, new aspects of the object may appear - the grey stone turns out to be more than just a grey stone.

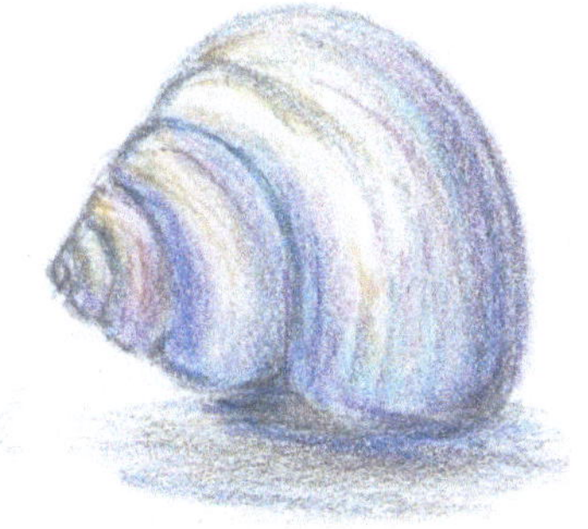

RHYTHMS IN EVERYDAY LIFE

A clearly structured day creates predictability and, in turn, security. In social therapeutic activities great emphasis is placed on the fact that every day has its recurring rhythm. Meals are at roughly the same time, and similar activities take place before and afterwards. Reading a verse before eating and giving thanks together before leaving the table can provide a clear beginning and end to the meal.

In many social therapeutic organizations residents and staff come together on weekdays in a morning gathering, shaped in various ways. Something significant happens in a person when the same ritual is repeated every day, e.g. reading a verse together, sometimes a different one every week or season. The breathing process is strengthened through simple and clear rhythms while the meaning of the words is gradually deepening. Repetition and perseverance have a strengthening long-term effect on one's own will. The repetition of the same thing day after day can awaken something deep inside us in the end, something unexpected which can gleam like gold once it is becoming conscious.

The week has its rhythm with recurring activities while the weekend and festive days provide a break from everyday life. For example, you can make a difference from workdays by putting a nice tablecloth on the table during the weekend or festive days, having a special breakfast and doing leisure activities.

The year also has its rhythm through the changing seasons and annually recurring festivals. It has the effect of recognition and security when the same festivals are celebrated in a similar way year after year, as described in the section on the festivals.

Many people with disabilities have difficulty with transitions and changes. It can be helpful to link certain festivals or other events to the naturally changing seasons. For example, when the winter clothes are put away, you can change the porridge at breakfast to a bowl of yoghurt to make it visible that there will be a change to a warmer season.

Setting up a seasonal table is a way to portray the changing seasons in the house. This is done by putting a plant or flowers and certain symbolic objects belonging to the season on the table. For example, in the winter a piece of white cloth be put on the table with white crystals or cotton wool for snow and in the spring, perhaps, some budding twigs and postcards of animals with their offspring. In autumn one could decorate the table with colourful leaves, chestnuts, and fruit and vegetables from the land.

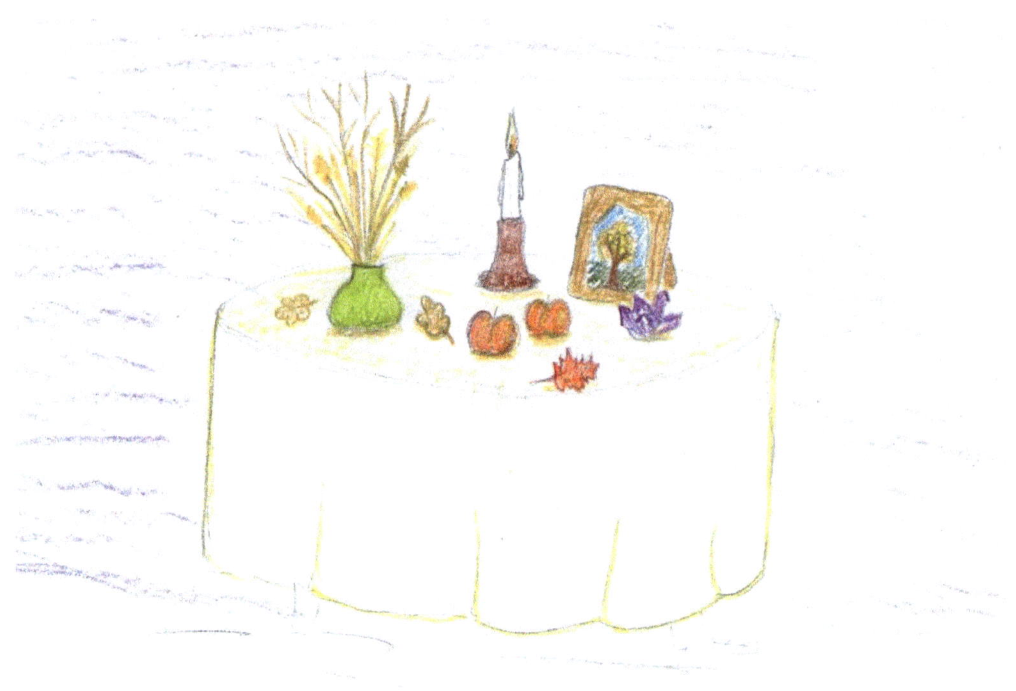

Seasonal table

THE FESTIVALS

The festivals of the year are important and are celebrated consciously and sensitively. Each festival stands for something special and by recurring every year it creates the effect of recognition, providing security and a personal connection to time. By celebrating festivals together in a group, a feeling of belonging begins to develop.

By understanding the spiritual background of each festival, it becomes easier to give shape and form to a celebration. The co-worker needs to understand the nature of the festival rather than just imitating how others do it. Then it will be possible for them to create a celebration more freely. Some effort is required to come to an understanding of the essence of the festival by familiarizing oneself with it and discussing it with colleagues. If you understand it better, you can become creative and find ways to keep the festival celebration alive and add new aspects from year to year.

For example: The Michaelmas festival, which (in the Northern Hemisphere) takes place around harvest time, is all about courage and strength. Muted, earthy, natural colours and seasonal vegetables fit better to this time than bright colours. Easter, on the other hand, celebrates the resurrection and new life and can be portrayed with light colours, tender greenery and symbols of returning life. 'Easter' comprises more than just the celebration of Easter Sunday. During the whole week leading up to it, Holy Week, one can turn to different themes for each day leading to Easter Sunday morning. Good Friday can become a day of introspection before the celebration of the resurrection.

QUESTIONS FOR REFLECTION:

HOW ARE RHYTHMS STRESSED IN MY PLACE OF WORK?

WHICH RECURRING FESTIVALS DO WE CELEBRATE?

WHAT KIND OF MOODS CAN I EXPERIENCE AT EASTERTIDE, FOR EXAMPLE?

IS IT DIFFERENT AT CHRISTMAS OR MIDSUMMER?

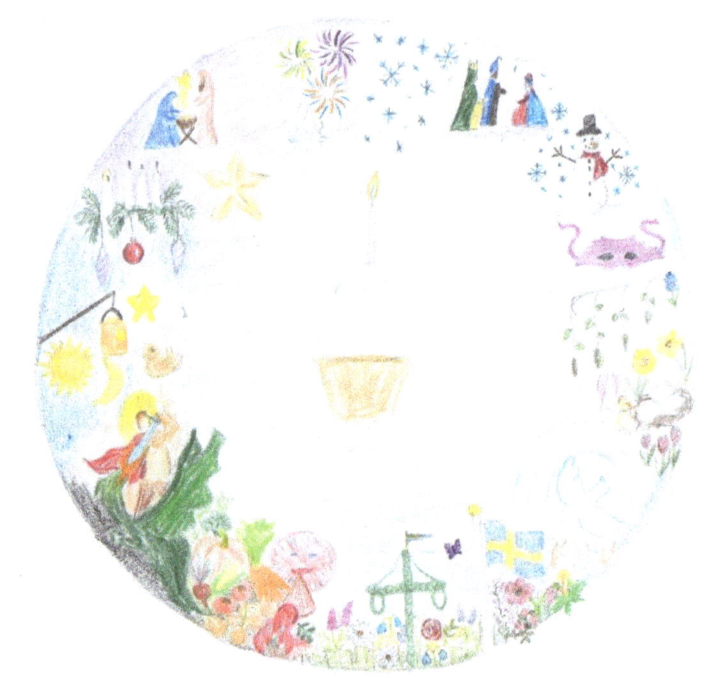

Examples of festivals which can be celebrated

The importance of work

A workplace is more than just a place where you go to pass the time and get paid. The workplace is an important social hub and perhaps the only opportunity for some to belong to a 'natural' social community.

As in all workplaces, it is important to feel needed and valued. Sheltered day-work places, or workshops for those with disabilities and challenges are places for those who are entitled to support to take part in daily work. It is the task of the support staff to create and provide meaningful work for those who take part. 'Meaningful work' is different for each individual person. Some people may need to do many different tasks and have things to do throughout the day. For others it might sufficient be to observe work being done and perhaps maybe to carry a compost bucket to the compost heap with the aim of assisting with the work there. Everyone contributes to the whole based on their own ability. An outside observer might have the impression that some participants in the workshop are not doing anything, but if you ask them at the end of the day what they have been doing they will let you know that they have done one or other job. They could have been present where workshop leaders and support workers were working on various projects enabling them to feel involved in the work. The workshop leader's presence and ability to have in mind those with special needs while doing the work determines the quality of the sense of participation.

Geert Mulders, an employee of a workshop in Telleby, Sweden, describes the role of work in social therapy like this: "... For us, it is not primarily a matter of providing a job, a daily occupation, but of placing the workers in a life situation in which they feel involved in the life of their environment..." (Liljeroth, 1994, p.97)

The workshop leaders make sure that those in the workshop have work they can manage well, but also give them opportunities for further development. They do this by creating possibilities suited to their individual strength. One creative supervisor can create work out of something which might cause problems to others. For example, there was a worker who tore paper into shreds all day. The support workers then came up with the idea to use these strips of paper as a 'backbone' for woven baskets.

Classical crafts have proved to be particularly rewarding work as there are clear and concrete results. The product will be something to use and benefit from. You can see how the candle you have been involved in dipping is lit in the evening; the bread you have been involved in baking is eaten with the soup, etc. The pathway from raw material to product is clear and can be traced back. It creates a feeling of being needed and can give professional pride: "Without me, there would not be any bread or any candles."

Here is another example: One worker embroidered irregularly and without any definite forms. The workshop leader then encouraged her to embroider small patches with colours that harmonize with each other. A colleague then sewed these patches together, so they formed a whole and became a beautiful picture admired by everyone. It is satisfying to have helped in a process and to have created something beautiful.

Why is it so important to bring meaning into the day? Meaningfulness, manageability and predictability are what make us humans feel well and cope with stress and challenges. These three factors provide a 'sense of coherence'. The sociologist Aaron Antonovsky researched this phenomenon and coined this phrase. (Antonovsky, 2005). The outcomes of the research into salutogenesis fit well with the basic anthroposophical ideas.

The creative aspect is also important in the work process, such as being involved in choosing colours, creating and making something new, being asked what you think of it and being given space to come up with your own ideas.

In addition to work, the workshop team is a social community where the workers can practice socializing and belonging. This is achieved by planning the work together, doing a slightly larger job in a group or in pairs. Then you will be the one who is missed when you're not there and welcomed back when you come the next time.

QUESTIONS FOR REFLECTION

WHY DO YOU GO TO WORK?

IN WHAT WAY IS WORK IMPORTANT TO THE PEOPLE YOU WORK WITH?

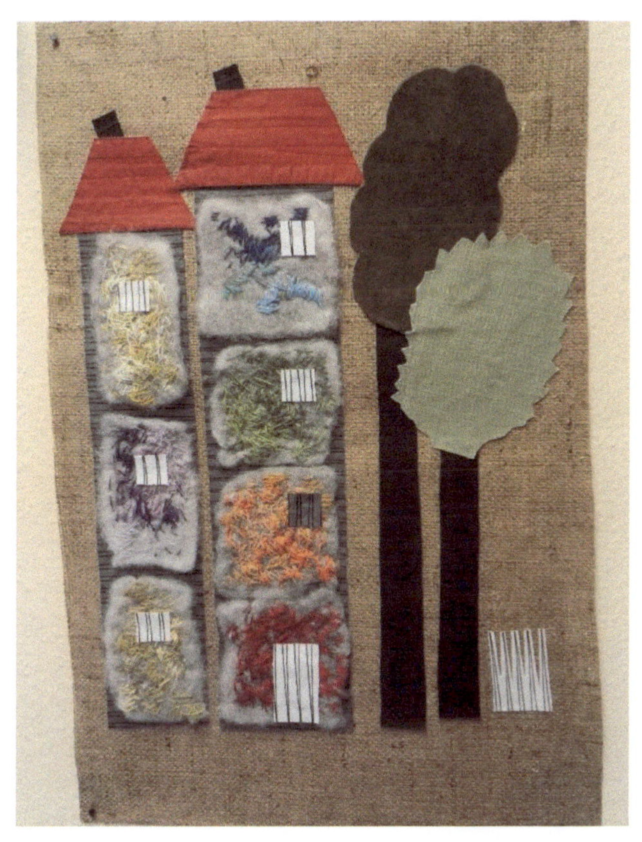

Board made of different parts

The concept of disability according to the anthropposophical image of the human being

The idea of reincarnation is that the ‘I’, which belongs to the spiritual world, is reborn. According to this idea, if there is an intellectual impairment it is the physical body, especially the brain which does not function as it should. On the other hand, the ‘I’ is always healthy at its core, even though it must be developed all through life. Think of a person with muscular dystrophy, spinal cord damage, cerebral palsy, or paralysis after a stroke. Behind any of these physical difficulties there is really no problem with intelligence. But sometimes we have a hard time perceiving this because our eyes see the physical body. It is similar with people who have intellectual challenges due to an impaired brain function. This can make it difficult to understand abstract concepts or cause autistic behaviour. People on the autistic spectrum have difficulties understanding feelings and behaviours in themselves or others. Despite any physical limitations, we all have a healthy inner core, the ‘I’. It is the individual personality which we can consider "healthy". This knowledge has an impact on the attitude with which we approach workshop attendees or behave towards them. When we have real human encounters from one person to another, it is not the physical body, but the soul and spirit we encounter. We meet and want to get to know the individual with his or her personality. Even if the person has a diagnosis, they are individuals and different from others with the same diagnosis. Even if a person *has* a diagnosis – (s)he her/himself *is not* the diagnosis!

As social therapists, we need to practice finding in others what makes them unique. A helpful thought exercise is to imagine what kind of person would stand before me if one were to "peel away" all physical impairments and difficulties from him or her. Which profession would he/she then take up? Which leisure interests would they pursue? What would be their strengths?

Starting from the idea of karma, we all have something to learn from each other. And it's not just that I, as a social therapist, teach something to the people I work with - I also learn myself. Maybe it's more the case that *I* am the one who must learn something if the encounter with the other person is a challenge for me. Then it can help to ask: "What can we do together?" and not "What can I do for this person?" One could also ask: "What is our common task?"

From the point of view of reincarnation, we are in some way involved in deciding what we want to achieve in our lives. One option for us could be to choose a life in which I need more support in the here and now - also to practice accepting help from other people and to be cared for. Everyone has the same value, regardless of whether they have chosen a life with or without the need for help.

What if the idea of reincarnation is true? Then I may be the one who needs extra help in another life. This attitude is reflected in how we meet and react to other people by addressing the healthy self and the potential for development within them. This also means that we do not judge or condemn people as having less value, because human dignity is not based on a functioning body. Knowledge of different diagnoses is fundamental so we can know what each person needs to feel safe and secure and to be able to communicate. It is just as important to see each person as unique and not just as their 'diagnosis' or 'syndrome'.

No two people with autism are the same, all have their own individual needs. On the other hand, we need a sound understanding of autism and other diagnoses, as well as working methods and methods that we carry with us in our 'toolbox'. We cannot expect a person to begin to speak if he has only learned sign language. A person in a wheelchair needs physiotherapy and a wheelchair to get around. We must adapt to the disability and *at the same time* perceive the individual. If one is allowed to develop professional and social skills, one can lead a more independent life. This is why it makes a difference to live in an environment where everyone's individuality is strengthened. The aim of social therapy is to create a social environment which enables the development of the individuality according to its own conditions.

QUESTIONS FOR REFLECTION

IF WE WOULD 'PEEL AWAY' DIAGNOSIS AND DISABILITY, WHO IS THE PERSON WE WOULD MEET?

WHAT WOULD BE THEIR INTEREST, PROFESSION, ETC.?

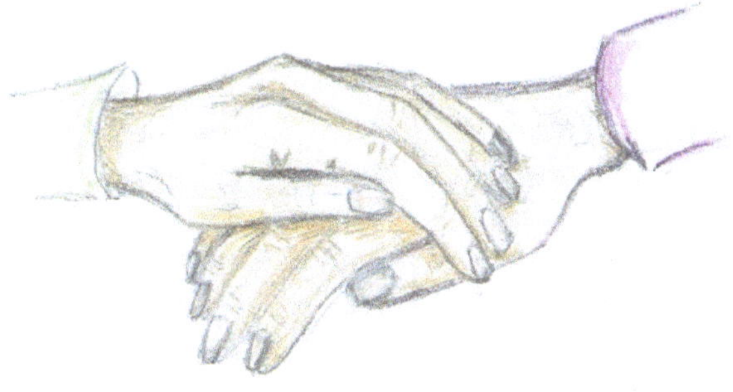

Helping hands

ENCOUNTER FROM PERSON TO PERSON

Social therapy is truly effective in interpersonal encounters. There we feel and understand with or without spoken words and can read each other's feelings and needs even if they are not communicated in words. To be truly healing it is necessary to look away from oneself and to approach the other person unselfishly, otherwise we risk projecting our own needs onto them. To be able to act in this way, it can help to leave our private "backpack" at home and put on "working clothes" when we begin our work. It is then important to be present in the here and now and to cultivate "devotion to the small detail." (R. Steiner in the Curative Education Course).

Social therapy is methodical, but it is not a method. If we look for a method instead of inwardly practicing spiritually, we risk losing our openness to the other in our encounter. One of the cornerstones of Anthroposophy is the nature of the human being and what it means to be human. By working on ourselves, we can also turn our feeling into a “tool" for the daily life. Intellect and intuition meet in the feeling. In this way, we can perceive the individual in the other person, but also use knowledge and experience to meet his or her specific needs. If we are open to the present moment, we can succeed in having genuine encounters. In every encounter, loving interest is a healing force. If we really care and are committed, we will discover new solutions.

We should enter the emotional state of the other person but behave with empathy without being absorbed in pity. If we are too sympathetic, we will transmit to ourselves the feelings of the other person and will no longer be free in our actions. If we are empathetic, we understand the feelings, but do not take them up ourselves. The antithesis of sympathy is antipathy. It causes us to have difficulties with someone and to keep our distance from them. The empathetic attitude is open and approachable, does not judge, withholds personal views and does not reinforce the emotional state of the other. Dare to listen actively, be open and hold back your own views. Dare to be open to accept things. Take the risk of showing your feelings, then you will be able to better understand other people's differences.

Another important tool in cooperation is humour. In fact, this may even be the most important tool. If we can laugh together, it can release blockages and build bridges over difficulties. Laughing together can create a relationship that can help us even in more difficult situations. On the other hand, we must not fall into the trap of laughing at someone, but we can try to laugh at ourselves and our actions. Dare to reveal a little bit of yourself! Keep in mind, however, that irony is a form of humour that is rarely understood if you have an intellectual disability.

Starting from the idea of karma, we can ask why we meet certain people. It is not so that I am the only one giving something to you. There is reciprocity to learn from each other. Or it may even be the case that I am the one who has something to learn from this encounter, especially if I experience the relationship with a person as challenging. Then it may be that I have to change or develop something in myself in order for the relationship to work. I can only change *myself* and not the other person. Open, exploratory questions about what happened may help to resolve the situation and improve relationships. Questions such as: What have I done? What happened? How can I do it next time? Ask this while focusing on what has worked. Test within yourself what you're doing and what you can do differently next time. Take time to reflect. It's not just what we do that matters. Our thoughts and attitudes also have an effect. If I find a starting point for changing my attitude to a situation, I can also change my actions. Whether we are more likely to connect or divide through what we say also influences our intentions and behaviour towards others. Thinking that a person is *having a hard time,* rather than thinking that he *is difficult*, deeply influences our attitude. We could also replace terms such as staff / clients/service users by terms such as coworkers/ residents/participants. There are not any specific anthroposophical terms that should be used, but in the organizations, one tries to use language consciously. Certain terms should be discussed with each other so that an awareness and consensus are created concerning which one to choose.

QUESTIONS FOR REFLECTION

HOW DO I ENCOUNTER OTHERS AND RESPOND TO THEM?

WHAT IS STOPPING ME FROM OPENING MYSELF TO OTHERS?

HAVE YOU MET ANYONE WITH WHOM YOU FELT ESPECIALLY CONNECTED, IN THE SENSE OF DESTINY AND KARMA?

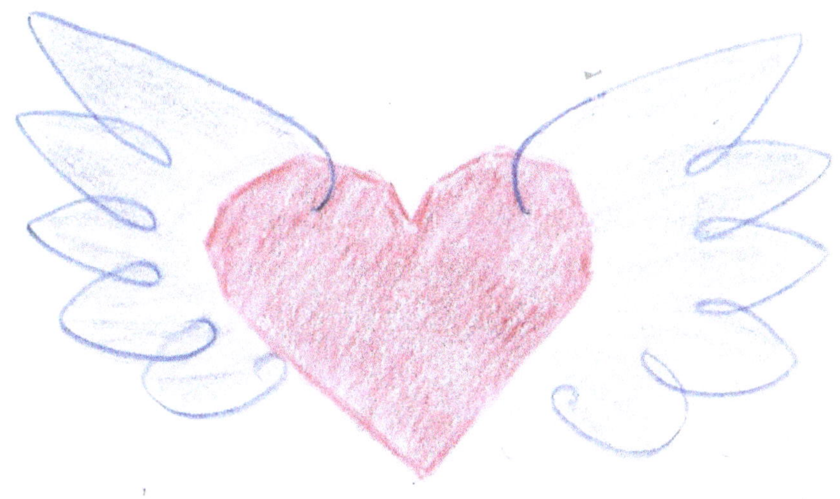

Work of the heart

INDIVIDUAL LIFE WITHIN AN COMMUNITY

Human beings are social creatures who depend on interacting with others to feel comfortable. Everyone needs the feeling of belonging to a social context. But the extent of someone's inclination to being social differs from person to person. Everyone must find a social context in which they can develop. One should be able to participate according to their own strengths and desires but also be able to experience development and inspiring encounters in an active community.

Social therapeutic activities provide opportunities for social community, for example in the group home where you can eat together, go on excursions together and socialize in common areas or at each other's homes. At work, there is social community in the group where the work is done in collaboration with others. You feel involved when you are at work, and you are missed when you are not there.

The experience at my workplace in Sweden shows that many people who move into social therapeutic housing initially have a strong desire for access to TV with many channels and other entertainments, but as time passes, they choose to be in the common areas and participate in the community and social life. There are many things on offer such as listening to music, talking together, doing craftwork or handwork, playing games, etc.

TV is not prohibited as one might assume. One could actually encourage watching a particular movie or entertainment program *together* instead of just having noise of the TV going on in the background.

There are opportunities to celebrate the festivals together for those who wish to take part. Then the festivals are properly organized and celebrated together with coworkers and residents. Everyone who wants to join should be able to participate on their own terms. For example, by participating in large joint celebrations for a short time only or sitting with a smaller group on the side for a while.

Arrange it so that everyone is comfortable. The social therapist's task is to help those they support to find the individual balance between the community and social life and being on their own and their personal needs.

QUESTIONS FOR REFLECTION

WHAT DOES MY OWN NEED FOR COMMUNITY AND BEING WITH OTHER PEOPLE LOOK LIKE?

CAN YOU IMAGINE A PERSON WHO HAS DIFFERENT NEEDS FROM YOURS?

CARING FOR THE ENVIRONMENT AND THE PEOPLE

If you go to different social therapy places, you are struck by the fact that, despite differences in the environment and the personalities of the founders, there is nevertheless something one can recognize, namely the atmosphere. Why is this? You can't make a checklist of what a social therapeutic place should look like. However, there is a desire to create something aesthetically pleasing with colours which make you feel comfortable and with consciously chosen materials. Perhaps you take inspiration from anthroposophical architecture and choose 'cut off corners' and gentle colours such as pink or purple. Natural fabrics are used in furniture, textiles, etc. where possible. The design is based on the idea of sustainability.

There is the desire to create both inside and outside something which is beautiful and not just functional. The idea behind it is to create a sense of homeliness and avoid an institutional character, while at the same time keeping the living spaces free from unnecessary items and clutter. Caring for this environment includes taking care of the entire surroundings. One could, for instance clean consciously, being fully in the present while wiping the table after a meal and thus practicing mindfulness.

The coworker needs to think about the small details. Setting the table beautifully, making sure that flowers in the vase are fresh and that there is order in the rooms. Also to have the right thoughts and feelings not to do mechanically what everyone else does. You could, for instance, think of putting a nice small tablecloth on the table, or lighting a candle. If someone has been away for a little longer, you might welcome them back with a bouquet of flowers or a few words on a card.

Concern for the environment extends beyond our immediate surroundings. We need to take responsibility for the whole earth in what we do, which is why there is an ecologically directed mindset in the choices we make. Based on this, we choose eco-labelled cleaning products, travel responsibly and do our best in using the earth's resources sparingly in general. Not everyone can do everything, but anyone can help improve the world in the small things.

In physical care, too, it is especially important that we do it thoughtfully, such as taking time to massage skin cream into the skin, brushing hair with a few extra strokes and paying extra attention when using the hair dryer. If someone is sick and needs a food tray in their room, it might be nice to bring a flower in a vase or to choose a special napkin or cup. It is important to nurture those around us and to have devotion to the small things.

THE IMPORTANCE OF DIET

As for nutrition, it is important to eat food that nourishes all the senses in addition to being nutritious and free of toxins. With this starting point, it speaks for itself that one would choose organic / biodynamic ingredients, and locally produced foods and seasonal vegetables, while eating less meat. We can do this, among other things, by buying food that has not been transported from far, such as tomatoes in the middle of winter, but instead making a salad with cabbage and carrots.

A meal nourishes both body and soul. In addition to the food itself, it is important to set the table nicely, eat together in peace and quiet and maybe have candles and flowers on the table.

It matters a lot how we prepare the food! A loaf of bread baked with care and love gives so much more to the person who eats it than a loaf prepared just to satisfy one's hunger. The same applies to all other meals, both in how we prepare them and how we create a pleasant mood at the table through everything from laying the table, being together socially and the mood which we create.

Avoiding gluten and milk protein may benefit some people. So-called gluten free/casein-free diets have been shown to have positive effects for some people with neuropsychiatric diagnoses. Gut flora is linked to our mental well-being which can be influenced by what we eat. Avoiding refined sugar and white flour, eating a varied diet with vegetables, whole grains, legumes and fermented foods improves intestinal health and in turn provides better mental well-being (Ekstedt and Ennart, 2017).

One needs to constantly update one's knowledge of what is good food for the body. The knowledge of what is good nutrition changes all the time as does the choice of available foods and thus what food we should choose for a diet which will help us feel well physically and mentally.

QUESTIONS FOR REFLECTION

HOW ARE YOU AFFECTED BY DIFFERENT ENVIRONMENTS?

DO YOU NOTICE A DIFFERENCE WHEN DOING A ROUTINE TASK BETWEEN BEING PRESENT IN THE MOMENT AND DOING IT UNCONSCIOUSLY?

Anthroposophical Medicine

There are different ways of looking at health. We often think that health is the absence of disease, and that illness and health are opposites. In anthroposophical medicine and care, health is more than the absence of symptoms. In the case of illness, the bodily balance is disturbed either physically or psychologically. The task of healthcare is not only to focus on the illness, but to strengthen the healthy aspects in the patient. The body can deal with minor imbalances such as colds through its self-healing forces. In more severe illnesses, the body needs help to heal through medicines among other things.

Due to the constant activity of the soul, health tends to fluctuate between two extreme conditions, for instance between diarrhoea and constipation. The healthy and normal lies somewhere in between. In either one of the extremes there is an imbalance which needs to be adjusted.

Anthroposophical doctors will try to see the whole person, body, soul and spirit (the self). They do not merely alleviate the symptoms but try to find their cause. The individual's experience of the disease plays a major role in diagnosing it.

Anthroposophical medicine often combines conventional medicine with natural remedies (integrative medicine) along with various artistic and other therapies. The life forces (ether body) are stimulated by homeopathic preparations, essential oils and herbs. In this way the body's own immune system is strengthened and can contribute to the healing of the illness. Anthroposophical natural remedies have been developed based on clinical experience and ongoing research of many years. Doctors who prescribe these medicines have the appropriate professional qualifications and are licensed.

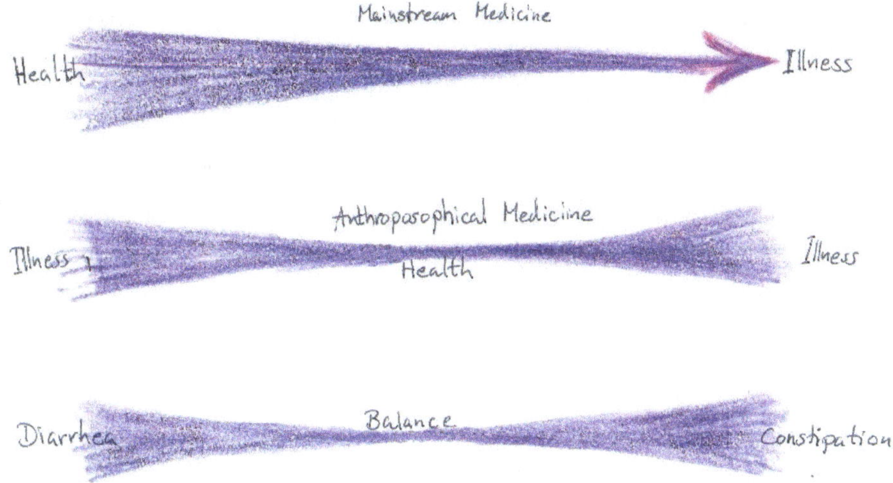

View of health

HOME PHARMACY

For mild illnesses, one can use anthroposophical remedies. This applies to minor injuries, small wounds, bruises or bleeding and simple colds. Remedies for these may be found in the home medicine cupboard after consultation with a doctor. In the event of more serious illnesses, you must always go to the doctor or the emergency department.

NURSING

Nursing and the use of home remedies are an important part of the healing process in addition to medicines and artistic therapies. A rhythmical foot massage with certain oils in the evening can reduce worry, anxiety and sleeplessness. A compress with herbs or oils is also a way to provide nursing care and relieve discomfort. Foot baths with essential oils or salt can also soothe or alleviate pain. Full body baths/ foot baths with mustard powder can reduce worry and anxiety as well as improve sleep.

QUESTIONS FOR REFLECTION

CAN YOU THINK OF A TIME WHEN YOU WERE SICK AND WERE LOOKED AFTER LOVINGLY, OR WHEN, ON THE CONTRARY, YOU WERE SICK WHILE BEING IN THE HOUSE ALL BY YOURSELF OR ON A JOURNEY?

THERAPIES AND ARTISTIC PRACTICE

Anthroposophical artistic therapy is different from conventional counselling therapy in that the various therapies aim to strengthen body, soul and spirit on a deeper level.

There are several forms of anthroposophical therapy, most of which are briefly described below:

- **Music therapy and Singing therapy** are based on the body as an instrument in which tones, intervals and rhythms work therapeutically. This therapy aims to balance sound, articulation and breathing. Vowels and consonants have different qualities which have as profound an effect on us as musical sounds and rhythms.

- **Eurythmy therapy** works therapeutically through movement while creating inner balance and supporting the body's own healing processes. The movements are based on the way speech sounds move in eurythmy and will either stimulate an opening gesture or a contracting one. The movements are made with the feet and/or the arms. The therapist does the movements together with the person who is receiving the therapy, adapting them to their individual needs and abilities.

- Through artistic creation in **painting and modelling**, the therapist 'reads' the individual and their constitution and then chooses appropriate therapeutic exercises based on the individual's limitations and one-sidedness. In this way opportunities are found for regaining balance in the soul. Various techniques are used such as painting with water colours on moistened paper, drawing with pencil or charcoal, modelling simple shapes with clay or beeswax. The aim is not to become an artist, but to work therapeutically.

- In **Oil Dispersion bath therapy,** full-body baths are prepared with essential oils. The warmth and activity of the oils are retained after the bath by wrapping the person in woollen material or thick towels without drying the body. Baths can relieve pain and be relaxing.

- **Riding therapy** focuses on the interaction between patient, horse and therapist. Collaboration with the horse strengthens the patient's self-confidence, exercises the ability to interact and communicate and increases initiative.

- **Bothmer Gymnastics** is a form of movement pedagogy that stimulates a dialogue between the person and their surroundings. It is a training to increase the ability to coordinate and orientate in space as well a sense for the whole body.

- There are two directions in **anthroposophical massage:** One according to Wegman/Hauschka and one according to Pressel. They both use rhythmical movements. The Hauschka massage is gentle and subtle, the therapist massages rhythmically with even movements. Pressel massage is a combination of deep pressure and rhythmical massage that is given alternately on the upper and lower body.

- **'Einreibungen'** [literally: 'rubbings' or 'embrocations'] and foot baths with essential oils can be applied by social therapists after an introductory training.

All anthroposophical therapies require long trainings in which theory and practice are interwoven. At the same time the student needs to do active inner work as well as study anthroposophy.

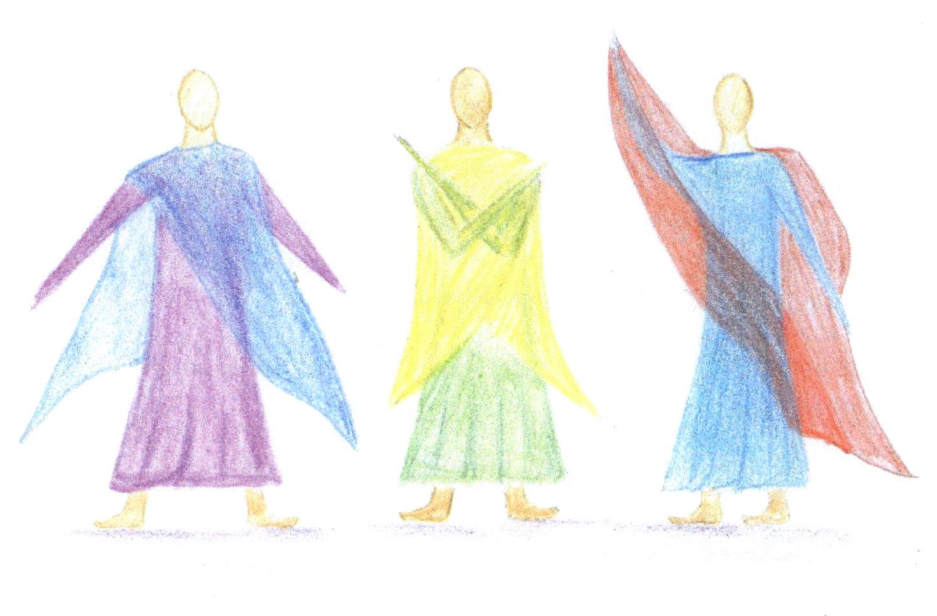

Eurythmy

CULTURAL EXPERIENCES

According to research, experiencing cultural activities together can alleviate depression, increase the quality of life and one's own well-being. It can reduce stress and strengthen the body so it can regenerate itself. Thus, culture is important in everyone's life. It can be seen from two sides: On the one hand one can actively be involved in cultural activity and on the other hand one can be the recipient of it. Cultural activity does not need to be complicated. It is important to enable people to be creative. Coworkers can, with initiative and enthusiasm, offer opportunities for creativity and activity: organizing a time for singing together, rehearsing a simple play for one of the annual festivals, reading a book aloud or encouraging those who are able to do so to write...

You can also paint, draw, write, write poetry, do hand work such as embroidery, knitting, crochet or much more.

Examples of one's own activities which are also activating:

Singing in the morning circle

Singing at annual festivals or other occasions

Playing and singing together

Practicing eurythmy

Folk dancing and circle dancing....

We can all be ***recipients of culture***. We can go to the cinema, theatre, concerts, exhibitions, museums. At home we could hang up paintings on the walls or listen to music.

There is a difference between culture and light entertainment. If it only brings about distraction, it will eventually drain our life forces, and if we consume it too often or for too long, we tend to become lethargic. Sustainably effective culture provides food for soul and spirit.

Questions for Reflection

How do I practice culture and creativity in my daily life?

In which form of culture do /want to take part?

Bonus questions as in the German and English version of this book:

Where and in which moments do you experience anthroposophical culture in the place where you work?

How do you get into dialogue with your colleagues about your questions?

Suggestions for Further Reading

English Literature for further reading:

Rudolf Steiner: *Education for Special Needs; the Curative Education Course*: 2014, Rudolf Steiner Press

Geertje Post Uitenweer: *Behavioural Disorders in Children and Adults: 2021: Temple Lodge Press*

Baars, Blomaard: *Good Care:* 2024, Temple Lodge Press

Rudolf Steiner: The Four Temperaments: GA57; Anthroposophic Press

Dr Gilbert Childs: *Understand your temperament.* 1995, Sophia Books

Robin Jackson (ed), *Holistic Special Education:* 2006, Floris Books

Pietzner, Carlo: A Candle on the hill – Images of Camphill Life. New York 1990: Anthroposophic press

Steiner, Rudolf. Agriculture Course (GA 327), 2014: Rudolf Steiner Press (Being republished)

Further Information:

Anthroposophic Council for Inclusive Social Development Dornach. https://inclusivesocial.org

APPENDIX:

The original Swedish version of this book:

Sara Sörgärde Siegers

Möjlighet till ett rikt liv

Wrå Förlag 2020

ISBN 978-91-985781-4-0

Excerpt p. 25 ff (from the chapter on the centres for social therapy in Sweden today...)

VÄRNA (Sweden's country organisation for curative education and social therapy)

has worked out the core values of today's curative education and social therapy institutions and summarised them in seven points.

The core values are as follows:

- the spiritual dimension according to our view of the human being

- the common thread in life

- individual life in community

- creative life and the importance of work

- mindfulness and respect for the individual

- Lifelong learning

- consciously designed environment

The specialist literature published to date is based on curative education (for children) and mentions in passing that social therapy is a form of curative education adapted for adults.

Ingrid Liljeroth (1994, p.12) also describes this in her research report and says that although social therapy uses the same knowledge base as curative education, it is adapted for adults.

. Here is her description of what curative education is:

- anthroposophy, with an in-depth view of the human being and a training path for staff

- an extended psychology that describes the course of life in 7-year phases and integrates insights into any obstacles to development

- Knowledge of how to organise these different phases of life in a holistically appropriate environment

- curative education methods and therapies such as teaching, eurythmy, Bothmer gymnastics,

speech therapy, music, therapeutic painting and handicrafts as well as the design of rooms and the immediate environment

- Medical knowledge

- Knowledge about the role of nutrition

A meaningful quote from Geert Mulders, an employee from the workshop in Telleby, describes social therapy: "...for us it is not primarily about providing a job, a daily endeavour, but rather to place the workers in a life situation in which they feel involved in the life of their surroundings. .." (Liljeroth, 1994, p.97)

Development of ideas: An idea or a thought can be both a formative force and a living organism in itself. The emergence of curative education and social-therapeutic institutions was based both an idea and a need. Even if an idea cannot be physically grasped or seen, its power forms structures to which physical reality can adapt. Liljeroth's report shows that in Sweden curative education and then social therapy were founded on the power of ideas and thought. Real need meant that both institutions and the conditions necessary for their establishment were created.

Liljeroth (1994, p.12) points to the overarching background of ideas, which I would like to include here:

1. the human being as a spiritually developing being. The disability is a link in the chain of this development process.

2. every human life is seen as meaningful and has a deeper significance.

3. starting from each individual situation, it is possible to create the conditions for development

4. curative educators and social therapists themselves have the responsibility to do everything possible for development.

This little book is intended to be and can only be a first introduction, a way to anthroposophy and social therapy.

(Translated from the German with DeepL.com and slightly adapted, ELF)

ACKNOWLEDGMENTS

Sara would like to thank all those who helped her by reading her drafts and making suggestions for improvements as well as making sure that this book could be published. Many thanks to her organization Ensjöholm, which allowed her to work on the book even in spare moments while she was at work.

My thanks in relation to the English version of this book go to Martin Schwarz for recommending that I do this work for Sara and for introducing me to her via email; to Lisa Grabsch for making a start to this daunting task, and a big thank you to Lisa Perry for proofreading the text with the eyes of a schoolteacher and a native English speaker (which I am not!).

And finally, thank you to Sara Siegers for writing this very accessible book with the lovely illustrations and for making it possible that it is available to all English-speaking social therapists, parents, siblings and anyone else who is interested in social therapy all over the world.

Edeline LeFevre

Northern Ireland